Mahamantra
Yoga

"Richard Whitehurst's *Mahamantra Yoga* is nothing less than a chalice of pure form that contains the elixir of highest truth. This book is magical, alchemical, and cut like crystal. It is a cleansing waterfall of light, sound, and spiritual resonance."

JAMES O'DEA,
TEACHER, AUTHOR, VISIONARY ACTIVIST,
AND FORMER PRESIDENT OF
THE INSTITUTE OF NOETIC SCIENCES

"*Mahamantra Yoga* is spiritually alive. Richard Whitehurst entwines practical guidance with authentic personal expression, thus encouraging the reader to fully embrace his or her humanness in the quest for spiritual enlightenment. This is a book for beginners as well as those who begin every moment anew."

JAMIE K. REASER, PH.D.,
AUTHOR OF *NOTE TO SELF:*
POEMS FOR CHANGING THE WORLD
FROM THE INSIDE OUT

"This book is a great companion for those of us on the path of chanting who want to go deeper into this very simple and extremely beneficial way of transformation and healing through the sacred Sanskrit sounds."

DEVA PREMAL AND MITEN,
WORLD-RENOWNED MANTRA AND
SPIRITUAL SONG ARTISTS

"*Mahamantra Yoga*'s potent combination of deep learning and profound personal insight sets this book apart. It is not only a valuable resource for students of meditation and mysticism but also an important contribution to contemporary spiritual literature."

STEVEN J. GELBERG, M.T.S.,
AUTHOR AND EDITOR OF *HARE KRISHNA HARE KRISHNA:
5 DISTINGUISHED SCHOLARS ON THE KRISHNA MOVEMENT
IN THE WEST* AND EDITOR OF *SRI NAMAMRTA*

"Richard Whitehurst creates a bridge for the modern Western reader to a world of wonders, powered by an ancient lineage and presently accessed through a very specific form of chanting. The principles that he so carefully presents alert one to what is needed for any path of inner development."

DAVID TRESEMER, PH.D.,
AUTHOR OF *ONE-TWO-ONE: GUIDEBOOK FOR
CONSCIOUS PARTNERSHIPS, WEDDINGS,
AND REDEDICATION CEREMONIES*

Mahamantra
Yoga

Chanting
to Anchor the Mind
and Access the Divine

RICHARD WHITEHURST

Destiny Books

Rochester, Vermont • Toronto, Canada

Destiny Books
One Park Street
Rochester, Vermont 05767
www.DestinyBooks.com

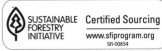

Text stock is SFI certified

Destiny Books is a division of Inner Traditions International

Library of Congress Cataloging-in-Publication Data

Whitehurst, Richard.
  Mahamantra Yoga : chanting to anchor the mind and access the divine / Richard
Whitehurst.
    p. cm.
  Includes bibliographical references and index.
  ISBN 978-1-59477-371-6 (pbk.)
  1. Mantras. 2. Spiritual life—Hinduism. 3. Yoga. I. Title.
  BL1236.36.W45 2011
  294.5'436—dc22

                                                              2011006836

Printed and bound in the United States by Lake Book Manufacturing
The text stock is SFI certified. The Sustainable Forestry Initiative® program
promotes sustainable forest management.

10 9 8 7 6 5 4 3 2 1

Text design and layout by Priscilla Baker
This book was typeset in Garamond Premier Pro with Florens and Albertus used
as display typefaces

To send correspondence to the author of this book, mail a first-class letter to the
author c/o Inner Traditions • Bear & Company, One Park Street, Rochester, VT
05767, and we will forward the communication or contact the author directly at
richardwhitehurst33@gmail.com.

To my dear godbrothers

Visnujana Swami, Aksobhya Dasa, and Aindra Dasa

A Note about the Roman Transliterations
of Sanskrit Words

The Sanskrit Devanagari alphabet consists of forty-eight characters: thirty-five consonants and thirteen vowels. The transliterations of the Devanagari script into the Roman alphabet that are given in this book are rough approximations only. It is hoped that this will give the nonspecialist reader an initial sense of the sound of the source materials quoted.

हरे कृष्ण हरे कृष्ण

Contents

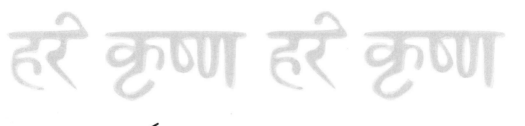

Foreword

By Edwin Bryant

The centrality of sacred sound is prominent throughout the entire history of Hinduism. From its very earliest origins, where the efficacy of the Vedic sacrifice depended on the perfect recitation of Vedic *mantras;* through the later Upanisadic period where the absolute Truth, *Brahman,* is equated with the sacred syllable *om;* and into later Hinduism where the great transcendent monotheistic deities all manifest their presence in their respective *mantras,* sound has encapsulated the highest foundational reality in Hinduism. It was thus a delight to encounter Richard Whitehurst's *Mahamantra Yoga:* what better testament to the timeless and transcultural efficacy and potency of sonic Hinduism than the testimony of an American adherent of a transplanted Krishna tradition in the West?

The *mahamantra* or great *mantra,* popularized in the West by the eminent Vaishnava teacher Bhaktivedanta Swami, was first propagated as a popular practice by the sixteenth-century Chaitanya, an ecstatic charismatic, considered to be Krishna himself by his followers. Perhaps no other tradition in the history of Hinduism has stressed and exemplified the theology and effects of chanting as much as did Chaitanya and his followers. While Chaitanya himself penned but a few lines, his followers wrote extensive hagiographies, theologies, and philosophical treatises featuring the Holy Name.

Richard Whitehurst has gathered together the more important of these insights and given us a glimpse at the psychological culture and attitudes conducive to successful chanting, which is nothing less than blissful and ecstatic love of God. The book is a wonderful little gem—well written, sophisticated in conceptualization, and spiritually revealing as well as inspiring. As a manual on chanting, the book brings together some of the important prescriptive guiding principles on chanting, written by some of the exemplary individuals in the Chaitanya tradition. Whitehurst thus provides us a very handy synopsis of Nam theology and praxis.

But where *Mahamantra Yoga* is unique is that it is written from an experiential rather than uniquely scholastic intention that is from an emic or insider rather than from just an academic frame of reference. So, in addition to its role as a prescriptive compilation of classical instructions of chanting technique, a user's manual so to speak, *Mahamantra Yoga* also provides an inspirational first-person narrative of the author's own chanting experiences. Thus, as a biography of sorts, we are afforded an insider's narrative of the practitioner's journey, encountering the author's own challenges and struggles over thirty-five years on the path of chanting, as well as a few accounts of the author's periodic successes—his attainment of states beyond the dualities of matter, and his taste, albeit brief, of the eternal, limitless, and blissful potential within the core of all beings. Indian meditation is experientially based—prioritizing direct perception—and it is important for Westerners to realize that they, too, are not incapable of attaining some of the experiences of which they read.

In this book, Whitehurst convinces us of the wonderful and universally attainable realities of the chanting process and the mercy of the Name. He reveals to us that chanting is a living and accessible process of self-realization accessible to us all even in our consumer-oriented day and age. And what was very welcome from an academic's perspective is that scholarly rigor is not sacrificed by this confessional perspective: the writing here is elegant and sophisticated, pointing to the keen penetrating insight of the mystic intellectual.

With *kirtan* and chanting becoming ever more popular in the Western world, I hope the book finds its way into the greater yoga community: I know no other publication that can serve both as a prescriptive manual of practice grounded in a time-tested Hindu devotional tradition as well as a descriptive record of experience that reflects the possibilities in our own day and age and Western landscape of encountering the bliss that is the most sublime of Divine personalities, Lord Sri Krishna, manifest as sound.

EDWIN BRYANT

Edwin Bryant received his Ph.D. in Indic languages and cultures from Columbia University. He has received numerous awards and fellowships and is the author of several books, including *The Yoga Sutras of Patañjali: A New Edition, Translation, and Commentary; Krishna: The Beautiful Legend of God; Śrīmad Bhāgavata Purāṇa, Book X;* and *The Quest for the Origins of Vedic Culture.* In 2001 he was appointed associate professor of religion at Rutgers University where he presently teaches Hindu religion and philosophy.

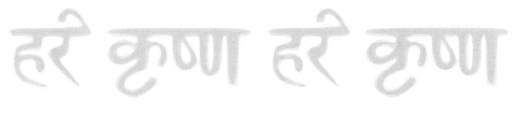

Foreword

By Charles S. J. White

I was very pleased and honored to receive the request from Sridhara dasa Adhikari (Mr. R. H. Whitehurst) to write a few introductory remarks to his new work, *Mahamantra Yoga*. I have read (and reread parts of) the manuscript and been touched by its literary and spiritual qualities. *Mahamantra Yoga* is both a technical treatise on the method of chanting the Hare Krishna mantra and a reflection on the author's own experience of the fruits of chanting. In many forms of the Indian spiritual life a sacred phrase such as the Hare Krishna mantra is recited over and over again in the pursuit of steadiness of the mind and access to the divine presence.

Hare Krishna Hare Krishna Krishna Krishna Hare Hare
Hare Rama Hare Rama Rama Rama Hare Hare

The specific mantra being used as well as the underlying theory of that mantra's recitation may be quite different from one philosophical and religious school to the next. Still, the outward manifestations of the practices remain essentially similar.

Sridhara dasa has written a treatise modeled on the ancient canonical texts of Vedanta. He has developed a number of *sutras,* or aphoristic phrases, in English that set forward the essential point that he is making about the method or fruits of chanting. He has written his own commentary to the sayings to expand upon their meanings. His observations are often very personal as he reflects upon the "realizations" he has known, as well as the problems of a psychospiritual nature experienced by devotees in general and the obstacles to the realization of the fruits of devotion to "Sri Nama Avatara," the personification of the personal presence of God in sound.

What is particularly compelling about Sridhara dasa's document is that it is the product of the devotional life of a contemporary Westerner, an American who has undertaken in a serious manner the spiritual path of *bhakti,* as introduced by his guru, A. C. Bhaktivedanta Swami Prabhupada, the founder of the Hare Krishna movement in the West. Sridhara dasa was initiated in 1972, and his training in bhakti included six years living in India. Of that time, half was spent in Vrindavana, the city of Krishna's principal *lilas,* or divine "games" with the cowherds and milkmaids, so charmingly depicted in the Bhagavata Purana.

Sridhara dasa is a householder devotee with wife and children. His mystical treatise testifies to the fact that one can pursue the goals of spiritual life in the midst of the conditions of work and profession in modern Western society. He acknowledges that the spiritual path is hard to follow in the secular society of the West; yet, whatever the obstacles, he is consoled by the divine presence, revealed in the recitation of the mahamantra. *Mahamantra Yoga* reminds us of similar works in the Christian spiritual canon, *The Imitation of Christ,* the writings of Brother Lawrence, and *The Way of a Pilgrim.* I personally rejoice in the fact that this new work has been added to the literature on the spiritual quest. It will prove its worth to devotees on the mystical path of bhakti as well as to students of the history of religions and Hinduism who are willing to take seriously the expansion of Hinduism to include outstanding devotees like Mr. Richard H. Whitehurst.

CHARLES S. J. WHITE

Charles S. J. White is professor emeritus of philosophy and religion at the American University in Washington, D.C., and has been a visiting professor and fellow in the Oxford Centre for Hindu Studies at Oxford University. He is the author of *Transformations of Myth through Time, A Catalogue of Vaishnava Literature,* and *The Garden of Loneliness: A Translation of Jayshankar Prasad's Ashu "Tears."*

हरे कृष्ण हरे कृष्ण

Acknowledgments

This book owes its existence to numerous sources. I have received knowledge, help, guidance, and inspiration from many well-wishers and friends. First acknowledgments must go to my *diksa* and *siksa* guru, His Divine Grace A. C. Bhaktivedanta Swami Prabhupada. He is that magnanimous personality who introduced me to Sri Nama Avatara. My gratitude to him cannot be known or expressed in some few words or paragraphs. May this book be the first written installment in my eternal and endless payback attempts to him for all that he has done and continues to do for me.

I offer my humble respects and heartfelt gratitude to the great pure devotee acaryas in this disciplic succession whose books and teachings have helped me in innumerable ways: Srila B. V. Narayan Maharja, Srila B. R. Sridhara Maharaja, Srila Bhaktisiddhanta Saraswati Thakura, Srila Bhaktivinoda Thakura, Srila Narottama Das Thakura, Srila Krishnadas Kaviraja Goswami, Srila Jiva Goswami, Srila Rupa Goswami, Srila Sanatana Goswami, and all the pure devotees of Sri Chaitanya Mahaprabhu who have come before and shown the way.

I am indebted to many godbrothers and godsisters for their help and contributions in the writing of this book. My godbrother Satsvarupa Dasa Goswami very kindly carried out extensive correspondence with me during the 1980s, offering numerous valuable suggestions that were incorporated into the text. His ongoing support and encouragement have been deeply appreciated. My godbrother Gargamuni Prabhu introduced me to my spiritual master and was the first one to assist me in hearing and chanting the holy names. To him I am deeply thankful and indebted. I am thankful to my godbother Narasimha dasa Adhikari who has given much editorial assistance as well as encouragement to bring the work to completion. I am thankful to Abhiram dasa Adhikari who has given help and guidance on many levels. I owe much to Jagatjivan dasa Brahmacari for his editorial assistance. There are many other dear godbrothers and godsisters, such as Bhakti Sudhir Goswami, Tamal Krishna Goswami, Vicitravirya dasa Adhikari, Subhananda dasa Adhikari, Yamuna devi dasi, Gunarnava dasa Adhikari, Vishalani devi dasi, and Tirtharaj dasa Adhikari who have given encouragement, help, advice, and inspiration. I sincerely thank all of them.

I would like to thank my good friend, wife, and godsister, Sevanandi devi dasi, who has sacrificed much and tolerated much during my pursuance of the writing of this book. She, more than anyone, knows my faults as a poor small living entity. I thank her sincerely and hope that this book will also further inspire her in her own evolution of mahamantra yoga.

Robert Lawlor, Duane Elgin, Arthur Deikman, Douglas Gillette, David Tresemer, Ronald Havens, Ernest Rossi, Robert Sardello, and my very dear longtime friend John Tresemer have all helped by way of advice, perspectives, and inspiration.

I am deeply grateful to my publisher, Ehud Sperling, and his excellent team at Inner Traditions International for their professionalism, expertise, and responsiveness in all areas of the production of this book. It is an honor to be associated with this remarkable publishing house and its people, including Mindy Branstetter, Kristi Tate, and Jon Graham. I also extend my thanks to my copyeditor, Jennifer Hope.

I am profoundly indebted to Professor Edwin F. Bryant for his extensive analysis of the text and his numerous and highly valuable suggestions for improving the manuscript and its finished structure. More than anyone else he provided the expert critical analysis that I had been seeking for so long. His incisive foreword will, I hope, assist the broader *yoga* community in its exploration of the realms of mahamantra yoga and thus perhaps find a deeper spiritual dimension to the variations of the more physically oriented practices of *asana* and *pranayama*.

Professor Emeritus Charles S. J. White, former chairman of the American University's Department of Philosophy and Religion, has honored this humble publication by his scholarly preface. May his words further open the minds of all thoughtful readers and intelligentsia who are new to the culture of mahamantra yoga and the path of bhakti.

I must also extend my warm appreciation to Professor Emeritus Norvin Hein of Yale University for his review of the manuscript and his helpful suggestions and advice.

Finally, I must not fail to mention the inspiration and guidance that I have received from Sri Nama Avatara Himself. He wanted this book to be written, and He has directed me, His tiny instrument, to write it. He has supplied the realizations—the substance behind the words of this book—and He has kept me connected to Himself even though I have repeatedly resisted. The great waves of *maya* may continue to toss this small life, dashing it upon the hard rocks of material frustration, but my true and meaningful direction will always be toward the glowing bowers of that bright realm of consciousness and spiritual flavor—the abode of Sri Nama Avatara. I have no other course. Thank you, Sri Nama Avatara, for showing me the way.

RICHARD WHITEHURST—SRIDHARA DASA
AHUALOA, HAWAII

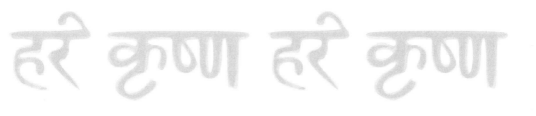

INTRODUCTION

The Internal Forest

Why this presentation? Simply to intensify and purify the individually and collectively applied culture of hearing and chanting the mahamantra. This presentation could be said to differ from others in that here an increased emphasis is placed upon the mystical domains of hearing and chanting—upon the *experiential*. This presentation is designed to orient one toward direct transcendental perceptions of both one's spiritual self and the spiritual nature of the mahamantra.

Chanting the mahamantra requires life. Naturally, the spiritually alive can chant with life. The spiritually alive are those who have passed beyond the superficial mechanical production of the apparent sound of the mahamantra and have become able (and enabled) to fuse certain spiritual conceptions into their chanting. The spiritually alive are those who have awakened to pure, transcendental, spiritual realizations. In hearing and chanting the mahamantra, purity is the force and realization is its substance.

Though extremely ancient, the dynamic, deep, and living process of mahamantra yoga was practiced and presented on a broad scale quite recently, some five hundred years ago in West Bengal, Orissa, and other parts of the Indian subcontinent by Sri Chaitanya Mahaprabhu, "The Golden Avatara," the infinite Personality of Godhead who adopted the role of a devotee of the Lord and taught bhakti-yoga, or pure devotion, to the Lord by personal example. Lord Chaitanya's movement of hearing and chanting continues to this day through His pure devotees. This movement becomes perceivable, meaningful, and overwhelmingly attractive to its beginning and intermediate followers when the power and mercy of Sri Nama Avatara (the living Godhead within the true mahamantra) enters within those followers' chanting endeavors. Then the mahamantra is no longer a "song" or "ancient cultural expression" but rather He is experienced as an unlimited, loving, personal being. He exists within the realm of utter truth and beauty, a plane that surpasses the shallow tidings of this material world. All who are sincerely endeavoring to advance in this practice must fight vigorously—relentlessly—to approach the platform of life in chanting. This tranquil, rapturous, and sacred subjective ground within our hearts is herein referred to (in its beginning stages) as the internal forest. Profound hearing and chanting of the mahamantra reveals the internal forest to the sincere souls who long to be there.

Sri Nama Avatara forsakes no one. Yet sometimes we forsake Sri Nama Avatara by a variety of inattentions while trying to hear and chant. Sri Nama Avatara waits for us in eternity, beyond our calendars and calculations, beyond the myriad variations of the insignificant course of our life. He is the cause of everything, yet He calls on each one of us with an abundance of pure love. We, His eternal children, must only hear His call.

Sri Nama Avatara comes to us through the favor of Sri Chaitanya Mahaprabhu and His followers, the most notable in recent times being His Divine Grace A. C. Bhaktivedanta Swami Prabhupada, my own spiritual master.

The realities and truths of the purely spiritual mahamantra are beyond the ordinary empirical methods of material comprehension. Persons obsessed by the limiting, relative worldview of material time and space cannot know Him. As long as a person considers the gross and subtle material bodies to be "self," that person, regardless of worldly title or position, cannot truly know what Sri Chaitanya Mahaprabhu's movement is. True and complete comprehension of Sri Chaitanya's movement of hearing and chanting the mahamantra eludes nearly everyone. Only the one who perfects chanting and hearing the mahamantra can know. Mundane sociological, psychological, philosophical, or comparative-religious approaches are of no avail. The movement of mahamantra yoga is in fact known only by internal, transcendental experience through the grace of one of Sri Nama Avatara's pure devotees. The *mahamantra* is the vehicle as well as the goal of this special type of transcendental experience.

So this presentation aims to help the reader move beyond ordinary material experience and attain genuine experience on the spirit-soul platform. The practices that are about to be presented do not pertain to the illusory material identity of any individual, whether racial or sexual. They do not pertain to the artificial geographical boundaries of nations on this remarkable planet drifting in the endless void of space. They do not pertain to the political or managerial organization of any institution. Nor do they pertain simply to the twenty-first century or to the fifteenth century or to any division or framework of conceptual time. Ultimately the principles relayed in this volume transport one beyond the illusory condition of durative time to the very foundations of personal consciousness . . . states of being that are dramatically different from the limited, dim, unfulfilling everyday consciousness.

One of the great *acaryas* of mahamantra yoga who taught by perfect example how to hear and chant, Srila Bhaktivinoda Thakura (1838–1914), divides chanters into two distinct classes. In his essay on mahamantra yoga titled *Nama Bhajan,* he says, "Some bear only the burden; others appreciate the true worth of things." Indeed many of us have felt all too often the oppressive weight of lifeless practice of mahamantra yoga. But we have also seen and felt the airy and intoxicating joy of that practice when the path was consciously and conscientiously pursued. We must ally ourselves with the second group . . . those who relish the mahamantra according to His value. We must remember that the mahamantra will begin to have immense and lasting value for each of us when we begin to perceive His transforming influence within our lives.

We must hear from the authorities of mahamantra yoga to understand the value of the mahamantra. And when we can incorporate that value into our approach to Sri Nama Avatara, by injecting into an intensely focused mind the higher conception of the mahamantra, then the mahamantra will actually begin to have significant and abiding value to us. At that time we will have established a spiritual relationship with Him, and our hearing and chanting of the mahamantra will have begun to enter into (and emerge from) our deep interior—our true spiritual being. Then we are vulnerable to Sri Nama Avatara's beneficent mercy, and soon there will be nothing more dear than the mahamantra, and the rays of His brilliant light will penetrate and illuminate the once dark regions of our hearts.

Nearly all who have heard the mahamantra are under varying degrees of misconception about the practice. With utmost effort we should now abandon whatever religious, psychological, historical, and cultural conditioning we may have regarding mahamantra yoga, picked up through contact with the so-called consensus reality and its various media. Let us try to begin with a clean slate. The mahamantra has nothing to do with relative conceptions of time and space.

Put simply, we are about to embark upon a process that takes us within ourselves—into the very deepest recesses of our innermost being. Soon enough, with practice and patience, we will enter the internal forest of the deep heart. Thus, by diving deeply within ourselves, we will begin to acquire a shining new perspective on the world about us and its original cause. Naturally, in our practice, we will begin on the "outside." The immediate starting point will be on the physical plane, and from there we will proceed inward to the mental regions and still deeper. For many, if not most, readers the aspect of self that now reads these words is not the true self. In fact, we will not really know who we are until the pure "I" is revealed to each one of us—at a glorious moment when our eternal, personal spiritual identity is clearly reflected upon the medium of the purified mind by a superior power. That superior power will appear to us as sound, and when that time comes, we will realize that the very sound upon which we have been meditating is not only "power" but also an unlimitedly loving being, the source of everything that exists.

This realization of the Supreme Absolute Truth through the chanting and hearing of the mahamantra is accessible to everyone. But even though the process is apparently simple and easily performed, it should never be considered merely mechanical. A mechanism or formula for approaching Sri Nama Avatara is given in this book, but the realization of Sri Nama Avatara does not ultimately depend upon any formula. Sri Nama Avatara is a person, and He takes the initiative to give direct revelation of His unlimited spiritual attributes to any living entity as He sees fit. Though acceptance of a bona fide teacher of mahamantra yoga is essential for advancement in its practice, on rare occasions Sri Nama Avatara Himself can bestow revelation of the spiritual plane even upon someone apparently outside the transcendental system of disciplic succession, or upon someone who has not followed the principles of sensory restraint and so is seemingly unfit for such revelation. Srila Rupa Goswami confirms this point in his *Padyavali*, text 29.

akrstih krta-cetasam sumanasam uccatanam camhasam
acandalam amuka-loka-sulabho vasyas ca mukti-sriyah
no diksam na ca sat-kriyam na ca purascaryam manag iksate
mantro 'yam rasana-sprg eva phalati sri-Krishna-namatmakah
[Translation:]

The holy name of Lord Krishna is an attractive feature for many saintly, liberal people. It is the annihilator of all sinful reactions and is so powerful that save for the dumb who cannot chant it, it is readily available to everyone, including the lowest type of man, the chandala (dog eater). The holy name of Krishna is the controller of the opulence of liberation, and it is identical with Krishna. Simply by touching the holy name with one's tongue, immediate effects are produced. Chanting the holy name does not depend on initiation, pious activities, or the purascarya regulative principles generally observed before initiation. The holy name does not wait for all these activities. It is self-sufficient.

Sri Nama Avatara is absolute and completely free to do as He wishes. Anyone may come under His influence. He is the ultimate controller. This principle is the same as the scriptural statement that "there are no hard and fast rules for chanting the mahamantra."

So this book concerns the approach to that supremely free personality, the prime objective for all living beings, the transcendental being who is the complete whole and the cause of all gross and subtle manifestations. Though the ignorant or uninitiated may superficially understand Sri Nama Avatara in the symbolic alphabetical form—*Hare Krishna Hare Krishna Krishna Krishna Hare Hare / Hare Rama Hare Rama Rama Rama Hare Hare*—He is far more than meets the eye. Let us keep in mind that Sri Nama Avatara is realized as transcendental sound vibration, and within the culture of mahamantra yoga our sense of sight is superseded by our higher aural experience.

For those who possess the simplicity and purity of mind to effortlessly hear and chant the mahamantra without offense (by not placing material conceptions upon the transcendental reality of Sri Nama Avatara), this volume may seem overly complicated and excessive in its treatment of the subject. To such pure devotees I offer my deepest respects. When dealing with the most sublime and holy names of the Absolute Godhead, less could be said and more could be said. May Sri Nama Avatara bless this humble effort.

Clearly this work is intended to serve only as a starting point in the culture of mahamantra yoga. The techniques presented here have worked well enough for me, but admittedly, they may not work for everyone in the same way. Some may have to find their own methods to fix the mind. This book presents the personal methods of just one insignificant practitioner of mahamantra yoga—one who by chanting and hearing the mahamantra has tried to follow Srila Rupa Goswami's order to "somehow or other fix the mind on Krishna." Practicing the following points will require much patience and attention. This book is definitely not meant for the mere acquisition of theory but rather for the transformation of consciousness through vigorous practice.

The highest states of transcendental consciousness obtainable through mahamantra yoga are not within my grasp at this time. Nevertheless I present the following work through the medium of my direct experiences and back up my ideas with the authoritative statements of *gurus* (the self-realized spiritual masters), *sadhus* (saintly persons), and *sastras* (revealed scriptures). I maintain the firm conviction that Sri Nama Avatara Himself inspired and directed much of what follows. The order of this presentation, the arrangement of the chapters and their points, surely is not absolute, but many of the specific points do indeed fall within the category of eternal, absolute principle.

Very briefly, something about the order of this book: chapters 1 through 5 guide the reader, step-by-step, into the various aspects of the practice. Chapter 6 gives descriptions of some of the early developments of the fruits of intensified hearing and chanting of the mahamantra. And chapter 7 summarizes the main body of the presentation in poetic form. An epilogue then offers some concluding words of a more personal nature.

There are four appendixes. The first gives the reader a contemplative practice for establishing a context for chanting. The second gives the complete listing of the aphorisms of mahamantra yoga. The third and forth list some of the broader principles of bhakti-yoga as well as the ten offenses to chanting. Serious application of this book's seventy-eight points, as well as regular study of the books in the bibliography marked with an asterisk, in the association of sadhus, will well equip the sincere practitioner for life's greatest adventure—the self's journey into the blissful region of the internal forest of the heart.

It is unfortunate but true that seldom do we find shining examples of prolonged nondistracted hearing and chanting. Indeed, mainly the opposite is observed. Many practitioners within the spiritual order have confided that, for whatever reason, their chanting has become a pale ritualized activity—and that aside from maintaining a vow, their chanting has little if any real perceivable relationship to their present life's spiritual evolution. The practical information in this book should benefit anyone serious about beginning—or re-beginning—the culture of mahamantra yoga. Certainly this book does not touch on all mistaken attitudes toward chanting, nor does it offer solutions for all circumstances. Nonetheless, be you a beginner or a re-beginner, may you glean something of value here for your culture of mahamantra yoga.

I confess that I am frail, flawed, and desperately reaching for the medicine of the mahamantra. May our spiritual preceptor, Srila Prabhupada, be pleased to accept this tiny soul's attempt to communicate various principles and realizations concerning the hearing and chanting of the mahamantra. This bit of writing is in no way meant to (nor could it) supersede Srila Prabhupada's own direct instructions on or glorifications of Sri Nama Avatara, now so nicely presented in *Sri Namamrta*. This is only an attempt to augment and further systematize the topics mentioned there, according to personal realizations collected during a period of more than twenty years as a large body of notes.

May we all deepen our relationship with Sri Nama Avatara and serve Him purely through His pure devotees. May we all come to know through direct experience much more about the limitless glories and powers of the mahamantra. This direct, personal experience of the transcendent Sri Nama Avatara is the final resting place for our hearts' most profound yearnings.

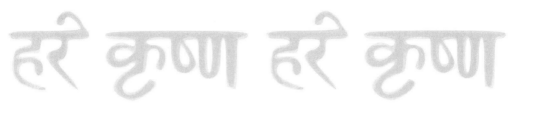

1 The Physical Foundations of Mahamantra Yoga

Helpful arrangements on the physical plane
immediately prior to hearing and chanting

Faith begins as an experiment
and ends as an experience.

PLOTINUS

Now we begin the actual practice of mahamantra yoga. The next five chapters will carry us, step-by-step, deeply into that practice. With care, intensity, and divine grace we should come to the experience platform of chapter 6. Mahamantra yoga will eventually deliver us to the glowing realm of realization—to the bright shores of the internal forest. So, with great seriousness at our command, let us now begin our intensified practice of mahamantra yoga.

Point 1.1
Eliminate all unnecessary sensory input or stimuli.

I am encased within a material body that is in turn situated within a highly distracting material environment. As the conscious observer I have connection to that environment through the senses of the body. Yet the fruitful culture of mahamantra yoga cannot evolve within an atmosphere of distraction, especially in the beginning stages. I wish to keep the mind highly focused upon the mahamantra in deep and abiding faith if I am to derive tangible benefit. As long as waves of sensory stimulation flood into the mind through the senses of the body, there is little hope of attaining intensified concentration.

I strive to understand that in a general sense my attention, my focus, and my generalized conscious awareness are of a distracted nature. Only when I understand this situation can I go about correcting it. Surely a diseased person must first recognize his disease before he can begin to seek a cure. Similarly, I recognize that my basic moment-to-moment conscious condition is one of sensory distraction. And then I seek to cure that distraction. Earnest and diligent action is required to establish a state of intensely focused attention upon the mahamantra devoid of all sensory interruption. Later, points 2.2 and 2.3 will probe the nature of sensory consciousness and my interlock with the plane of time and space. This information will help me overcome the bondage of mundane sensory stimulation while hearing and chanting the mahamantra.

Point 1.2
Establish an environment and time for practicing mahamantra yoga.

Environment
In the beginning there is a requirement to establish an environment truly favorable to the practice. I should find a calm and quiet place, free from the possibility of sudden disturbances. Locked doors might be necessary. Notification of others might be required. If possible there should not be extreme heat or cold. The place should be clean and orderly to soothe my passage through the various psychological and emotional

planes on the way to the pure hearing and chanting of the mahamantra. In his *Govinda Bhasya* commentary on the *Vedanta-sutras,* Srila Baladeva Vidyabhusana points out that though most people consider places of pilgrimage ideal for meditation, even in such places there can be grave distractions. In his commentary he cites a passage of the *Sruti-sastra* that states, "mano'nukule," one should meditate "where the mind feels 'favorable.'" This is obviously a matter of individual contact with a particular setting that either does or does not support an inward turning of the attention.

Cats, dogs, insects, and especially other human beings should not be present during my private practice of mahamantra yoga. Though total isolation from human society is not advocated here, few could argue that there is anything more stimulating or distracting than another human being. When attempting to chant the number of rounds prescribed by guru, I might have to arrange with family members, friends, or associates to leave me alone during some designated portion of the day—a time considered sacred by me.

A further note should be made here. Sometimes I may feel that having the company of others who are also engaged in the culture of mahamantra yoga is a favorable circumstance for progress. Indeed the association of sincere practitioners of mahamantra yoga is a principle of utmost importance. But let me clarify the issue. The relationship with Sri Nama Avatara takes on primary importance during the practice of hearing and chanting. If I can have the association of completely pure devotees of Sri Nama Avatara, then that opportunity should not be missed under any circumstance. However, there is no great benefit gleaned through the direct association of other devotees during my private hearing and chanting, or *japa.* Naturally, peer-group approval should not play a role in my culture of mahamantra yoga, not to mention the need for company to keep me from falling asleep. (Countering sleepiness will be taken up in point 1.5.) *Kirtana,* the congregational hearing and chanting of the mahamantra, is obviously a different issue because it necessarily requires other persons for its execution.

Time

The very best time for practicing mahamantra yoga is the period between midnight and sunrise, especially one to two hours before sunrise. The reasons go from obvious to obscure as to why this time is best. Most people sleep at this time preceding sunrise; so do most dogs, cats, birds, and nearly all other species that can disturb or make noise.

Other more subtle characteristics exist at this time. First, the very fabric of the mental plane rests in a passive state during these hours. The *sattva-guna* predominates, and the mind is in its most placid, tranquil, and composed condition. The sincere student of mahamantra yoga should take advantage of this circumstance. I must devise a personal schedule and stick to it. "Early to bed, early to rise" has proven a useful adage.

Second, a vast cosmic theme takes place daily during the predawn hours, and the conscious or unconscious perception of this theme can be used to one's advantage. The great eye of God, the sun, the abode of the plenary expansion of Sri Krishna—Lord Narayana as Hiranmaya—is soon to make His appearance. The Supreme is about to enter into manifestation before me. This fact is confirmed in the *Srimad-Bhagavatam*, Fifth Canto, chapter 7, texts 13 and 14. No other segment of the twenty-four-hour cycle is nearly as powerful psychologically speaking as these predawn hours. This theme runs parallel to the realization of the full appearance of Sri Nama Avatara in His limitless glories. "The Supreme Personality of Godhead is about to advent Himself—the dawn is breaking."

It does not matter whether I am conscious or unconscious of this theme, it will act just the same. Variations in the weather or the changes of season affect my mood and my attitude toward life and the world. Similarly, when the light of God is about to enter my life from the cosmic perspective, my mood and attitude are altered favorably, especially when my intention is to commune with the Supreme by hearing and chanting His transcendental names.

As I deepen my realizations of the mahamantra there is a strong tendency to hear and chant for longer periods of time regardless of the situation of the sun in relation to the earth. The transcendental sound seeps into the very fabric of life and barely a minute will pass when the mahamantra is not being heard—cleansing the mind and pushing me into deeper and deeper states of transcendental ecstasy.

Point 1.3
Free the environment from external distractions.

As a student of mahamantra yoga I should become aware of my immediate environment and make all possible adjustments to minimize distractions. Distractions could include dripping water, whistling air currents, ticking clocks or wristwatches, and so on. Distractions could also include, for instance, excessive heat or cold, excessive light or darkness, or excessive lavishness or starkness of the setting. I will be on guard, although I will not be obsessive. I will do my best to create a mild, neutral, and meditative situation. As I advance into higher and more detached states of consciousness, I will notice that the various sensory elements that make up the external reality begin to fall away and lose prominence. As I begin to enter into the mode of ceaseless hearing and chanting of the mahamantra, the environment will not matter for at that time Sri Nama Avatara and not sense perceptions will dominate the field of consciousness.

In his *Sri Harinama-cintamani,* Srila Bhaktivinoda Thakura discusses this topic of sensory distraction quite strikingly. In the twelfth chapter, titled "Pramadah," Srila Bhaktivinoda remarks:

Pramadah means inattention or carelessness. It is from this offence that all *anarthas* arise. The wise men recognize three types of inattention: indifference, inertia, and restlessness. If inattention is present in one's chanting of the Name, one cannot attain nistha or steadiness; and without steadiness one cannot attain *prema* [pure unalloyed love of God]. Even if one successfully overcomes all the other offences in chanting, and even if one chants the Name continuously, *prema* may still not appear. The reason for this is that one is committing the offence known as *pramadah* or inattention. This offence will block the progress to *prema*.

The first type of inattention is indifference. Indifference is a lack of interest in the Name caused by a strong taste for material things within the mind. The first remedy given for indifference is to take the association of a pure *Vaisnava* who is properly chanting. Bhaktivinoda Thakura continues:

> In a secluded place, one should chant the mahamantra in his company for a short time (a few hours) each day. By seeing that *vaisnava's* attraction for the Name, one will become inspired to give up indifference. Gradually the mind will become fixed on the mahamantra, and will always be hungry for the nectar of the mahamantra.

If there are no pure devotees present to directly associate with, I may then resort to another method to overcome indifference. Bhaktivinoda Thakura goes on to further explain:

> Another remedy customarily used by the devotees is to isolate oneself and cover all the senses. One may carefully chant in a room by oneself with the door locked (to avoid interruption from others), or cover the eyes, ears, and nose with a cloth or anything serving that function (in order to prevent exterior stimuli from distracting the mind). Making the mind concentrate on the mahamantra in this way, one will quickly develop steadiness (*nistha*) throughout and then attraction (*ruci*) for the Name. In this way the fault of indifference will be surpassed.

Inertia, the second form of inattention, is characterized by a lazy attitude—"slow to start, slow to chant." Bhaktivinoda Thakura throughout points out:

In this state of mind, even when one manages to chant the maha-mantra, one always seeks respite or opportunities to interrupt the chanting. Again, the remedy for this is to take association of the *vaisnavas*. The *vaisnava* [pure devotee] always thinks that he should not waste his time on other activities. With this in his mind, he constantly chants japa of the mahamantra, experiences the nectar of the mahamantra, and desires nothing else. One should seek out such *vaisnavas,* and seeing the example of such diligent Krishna consciousness, one will be inspired to follow in their footsteps and give up the lethargic mentality.

Bhaktivinoda Thakura further mentions:

One will develop admiration for their quality of not wasting time. In his mind he will think, "When will I be fortunate enough to chant and sing the mahamantra as these *vaisnavas* do?" By this inspiration, enthusiasm will replace laziness, and the person will overcome the offence of inertia in chanting the mahamantra. He will become determined to increase his number of rounds. By the mercy of the *vaisnavas, vaisnava* italicized throughout his mind will become extremely eager to chant and increase his chanting, and the offence of inertia will soon be gone.

The third type of inattention is described as restlessness, and it requires a major effort on the part of the spiritual aspirant to overcome this stumbling block. Restlessness becomes manifest when desires for wealth, sexual partners, material success, and recognition are present within one's consciousness. The remedy for restlessness is association with pure *vaisnavas,* hearing from them, and also strict observance of *vaisnava* behavior. These topics of association with *vaisnavas* and *vaisnava* principles are mentioned in appendix 3 of this book, and these topics can be further studied in the various devotional books listed in the bibliography.

Point 1.4

Wear clothing that does not produce distractions or emphasize the configurations of the body.

My identification with the body and its tactile sense runs deeply through my psyche, and I attempt to take measures to reduce this distracting situation. Because clothing stimulates the tactile sense, it is necessary to find that style and fabric that will reduce my awareness of these sensations. The clothing should allow the skin to breathe and should not stick to or irritate the skin. Clothing produced from artificial man-made fibers causes perspiration and itching sensations and so will be found to be distracting. It should be avoided. Loose-fitting clothing of a pure natural fiber such as cotton, linen, or silk is best for wearing in the practice of mahamantra yoga.

For those with male bodies either a *dhoti* or loose-fitting pants will be suitable for covering the lower portion. The upper portion may be covered with a *kurta* shirt, t-shirt, or with a light *chaddar* (wrap). For those with female bodies a loose cotton dress, yogi pants and *kurta* shirt, or a *sari* will be suitable.

There are distinct advantages to having the body covered, as opposed to having the body uncovered. The illusory identification of self with the material body is reinforced when the untrained conditioned self sees and contemplates the bodily limbs. To set an example for his disciples Srila Bhaktisiddhanta Saraswati Thakura made it a practice never to look into a mirror. The projection of consciousness outward into material space, evoking the feeling of material hands, arms, legs, feet, and head, is all part of the great illusion of material consciousness. I will never know Sri Nama Avatara as long as I cling to this illusion—to the lake of sensation known as the material body—a thing completely different from what I really am.

As sex attraction is one of the most powerful factors contributing to false bodily identification, it is only fair to the opposite sex that one dress in such a way as to de-emphasize the configurations of the body, specifically at times when one participates in the congregational practice of mahamantra yoga.

Point 1.5

In a mood of utmost seriousness and intensity, regulate the unlimited variables of bodily movement and posture through the authorized techniques of dancing, sitting, and moving the beads.

Physical survival and sensory fulfillment necessitate bodily movement. But by its very nature, bodily movement is distracting. There are two major kinds of mahamantra yoga: private (*japa*) and congregational (*kirtana*). In both, bodily movement should be carefully controlled.

In the chanting of *japa* the basic seated yoga postures along with the *mula-bhanda* (contraction and drawing up of the anal sphincter) will prove highly effective. Though difficult at first, keeping the back perfectly straight for the duration of my hearing and chanting period will also prove highly effective as my days progress toward more profound realizations. These observations are confirmed in the Bhaktivedanta purports to *Srimad-Bhagavatam* 3.28.8: "Sitting in an easy posture is called *svasti samasinah* . . . that posture will help one to concentrate his mind on the Supreme Personality of Godhead." Therein it is also mentioned that a straight back will keep one from falling asleep. Sleep is certainly a great destroyer of both physical and mental posture. The practices of *mula-bhanda,* reduction of eating, not eating after sunset, eating only light foods, and taking sufficient rest will also assist in keeping body and mind alert for hearing and chanting. Texts on *hatha-yoga* can supply details on the easiest ways to assume both *mula-bhanda* and also the ideal sitting posture.

The sitting postures with locked or slightly locked legs will be found to build a stronger psychological base of steadiness than those postures that give greater scope for movement. Though standing perfectly still might allow some freedom from distraction, standing also gives the greatest scope for whimsical movement from place to place. We find a remarkable statement in the *Vedanta-sutras,* fourth *adhyaya,* first *pada, adhikarana* VI, sutras 7–10:

asinah sambhavat

[Translation:]

> Let him recite the Name of the Supreme Godhead in a sitting posture, [for prayer and meditation are] possible in that posture only.

As I move closer to Sri Nama Avatara I will gain the power to sit totally erect and motionless for very long periods. I start with a specified short span of time and gradually build up. The mind will urge me to get up and walk about. The mind will tell me to slouch while sitting. The mind will tell me to open the eyes and look about. The mind will dictate so many things. I will observe all of this and then ignore or neglect the whims of the mind, knowing these random thoughts to be mere mental clouds that will float away in due course. It is generally not easy in the beginning, but what thing of value ever comes without a vigorous, concerted effort?

A firm slightly padded sitting surface is ideal. Either smooth carpet, a piece of firm foam padding, or a folded blanket will work nicely.

Chanting outdoors, pacing, moving, and looking about, "*japa* walks"—these will bring about a highly distracted state of mind and are to be avoided during those times in which I am endeavoring to fulfill a numerical vow on the beads. I should sit down firmly when employing the chanting beads. And with the right hand I should hold the beads near the body (but not touching it), cocking the lower right arm at a ninety-degree angle in relation to the torso and upper right arm. Each bead is to be rolled between the right thumb and middle finger as the complete thirty-two syllables of the mahamantra are being chanted. This process is to be followed on each of the 108 chanting beads that make up the *japa-mala* rosary. This will take between six and ten minutes and is commonly referred to as "chanting one round." Sixteen rounds per day is a recommended minimum amount of private hearing and chanting for those who have been initiated into the tradition. For beginners three to four rounds would be a good place to begin.

While chanting, the left hand should remain motionless and should be situated so that the fingertips are minimally stimulated. Banging the beads, shaking the beads, resting the beads on the feet or the floor, employing small metal counting devices—all of these methods may be considered nonprogressive. The beads are not to be viewed as some variety of alarm clock or witch doctor's juju rattle. I try to maintain control, reverence, and sobriety when touching and moving the beads. I should wash the bead bag regularly.

Movement during the congregational chanting of the mahamantra should assume the stately dance of crossing one foot before the other to the rhythm of the three-beat *kartala* playing. Or I may stand still with hands folded. Wild jumping and whirling should be reserved for times of deep and utter absorption in the sound vibration of the mahamantra—a stage when my feet, legs, and body are moved about ecstatically by Sri Nama Avatara Himself, not by any facet of my ego, which is so often prone to seek adoration and praise. This wild-dancing mode is a later stage in the culture of mahamantra yoga.

In a mood of humility and devotion I should first concentrate on hearing and chanting during *kirtana* with closed eyes. I should not concoct new dance steps that have never been demonstrated or approved by the pure devotees of Sri Nama Avatara. This topic is discussed in the Bhaktivedanta purports of the *Sri Chaitanya-caritamrta, Adi-lila,* chapter 7, text 88, wherein it is stated:

> Sometimes persons who have no love of Godhead at all display ecstatic bodily symptoms. Artificially they sometimes laugh, cry, and dance just like madmen, but this cannot help one progress in Krishna consciousness . . . If one who is not yet developed imitates such symptoms artificially, he creates chaos in the spiritual life of human society.

And elsewhere in that chapter's purports it is further stated: "If one chants the holy name of the Lord just to make a show, not knowing the secret of success, he may increase his bile secretion, but he will never attain perfection in chanting the holy name."

Point 1.6
See to cleanliness, order, and symmetry of the external environment and physical body to foster a favorable mental environment for Sri Nama's appearance.

Point 1.6 is a summary of the first five points, and it leads us to the gateway of the mental plane. As with environmental cleanliness and order, bodily cleanliness is essential to attain to the states of concentration necessary for tangible advancement in mahamantra yoga. A clean body soothes and calms the sensory systems. I will bathe regularly and try to cleanse the body just prior to the time that I have set aside for hearing and chanting. I will notice a feeling of freedom within the mind after all impurities have been washed from the surface of the body. This is another instance of symbolic advantage that can be used to foster progress. A clean body is reflected into the mind and causes thoughts of cleanliness. A clean mind is a suitable receptacle for the appearance of Sri Nama Avatara.

Before chanting and hearing the mahamantra I should thoroughly clean the mouth as well. The teeth can be cleaned with a conventional toothbrush and dentifrice. If the lips are dry I can apply a lip balm or moisturizer. If required, I should evacuate the bowels and empty the bladder. Bathing should be the last of the items to be undertaken. I should turn all these practices into a routine so that the physical foundations of mahamantra yoga take place automatically. Then I will be properly prepared to acquire the mental foundations of my mahamantra yoga, the subject of chapter 2.

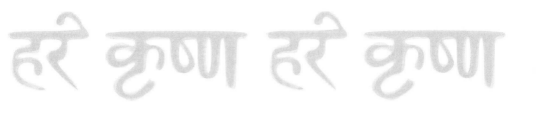

2 The Mental Foundations of Mahamantra Yoga

Helpful mind-postures, attitudes, and meditations to be executed immediately prior to hearing and chanting

The means of getting there are the same as the qualities of being there.

LAZARIS

Point 2.1
Offer obeisance to the spiritual master, the living example of pure hearing and chanting—the perfected mahamantra yogi.

I cannot approach the Absolute Truth in His sound-vibration manifestation directly. Approach to Sri Nama Avatara is possible only through the transparent via media—the pure devotee of Sri Nama Avatara. Therefore, I will first acknowledge the spiritual master and with all humility and gratitude offer respectful obeisance to him. Also I try to regularly read the authorized books that deal with this topic.

Point 2.2
Stabilize mental flux and turn consciousness inward by the brief exercise of establishing presence of self in the heart, regulating the breath, and focusing awareness on the inner field of vision.

Here is a simple mechanical process of a nonabsolute nature that can fix the mind and direct the attention from its distracted outward-turned mode, called *paranga-cetana* in yogic terminology, to its inward-turned meditational mode, *pratyak-cetana*.

I sit quietly in my easy posture and begin regulating the breathing by counting. I set a number that is attainable for my lung capacity. The "square" breathing pattern is simplest and should work well enough for most people. I close the eyes and commit to keeping them closed for the duration of my chanting of the mahamantra. Counting mentally I keep breathing in through the nose to the point of mild fullness of the lungs, and now I note my *number*. I hold the breath for that same count, exhale smoothly and quietly through the nose for that count, and then hold the breath outside for that count. I patiently repeat the process. After some five to ten repetitions I notice a marked change in the character of the mind. Its flickering and unsteady quality begins to be replaced by a calmness and serenity. This practice is mentioned in the *Brahma-vaivarta Purana,* and it is nicely recounted in *The Nectar of Devotion,* chapter 10, wherein it is stated:

> These breathing exercises are meant to mechanically fix the mind upon a particular subject. That is the result of the breathing exercises and also of the different sitting postures of *yoga.* Formerly, even quite ordinary persons used to know how to fix the mind upon the remembrance of the Lord . . .

As the mind calms I focus my inner "looking" upon the dream field or screen—that place within the mind upon which the play of dreams takes place. I look *inside* from the heart in a relaxed way as though gently trying to see into the depths of my inner visual field. As I perform these three actions—breathing, counting, and looking from the heart upon the dream field—I begin to notice a pronounced shift in the orientation of consciousness from its usual outward-turned sensory mode to a new and far more suitable inward, centripetal orientation. With practice this reorientation is accomplished easily within thirty to sixty seconds. Now the field of the mind is ready for planting the various seeds necessary for fruitful mahamantra yoga.

Point 2.3
Consider the gateways between the conscious self and the external world. These gateways are the five sensory systems.

I must read this section slowly and thoughtfully to catch its significance and value. Once I have understood this point, recalling it will consume no more than one to five seconds. The purpose will be to diminish the false identification of the self with the body. Chanting the mahamantra while maintaining the false identification of body as self is as effective as trying to start a fire while pouring water upon the wood. As Srila Bhaktisiddhanta Saraswati Thakura mentions in his essay "The Nomenclature of the Absolute": "If we think we are mind and the external body, the Transcendental Sound will have no effect on us."

By giving consideration to point 2.3 before engaging in the hearing and chanting of the mahamantra, I concede, "I am not this material body, nor am I the body's perceptions. In fact the perceptions of the body and my conceptions about the perceptions of the body are a major source of my illusory misidentification of self as body. I reject the illusory nature of my sense perceptions, as well as the false identification that I am this material body." I should carefully and patiently think through the following points and reread when necessary.

As might be expected in the realm of dualistic consciousness, there are two orientations for the conditioned soul: the external world of apparently tangible objects and the internal world of subjective experiences. The external reality is the fantastic gross-material plane that roars on all about me. It is that which I perceive to be outside of my body and within which I find my body situated. The internal reality is the world of perception and observation—the dimension of witnessing, which is apparently limited to the boundaries of the bodily sheath. For the purposes of this discussion of the preliminary practice of mahamantra yoga, the self may be said to lie at the very center of the internal reality. When I am obsessed with the outward-turned consciousness, there is little if any attention paid to the internal reality, though it is the more essential ground of my being. In those instances I am involved in looking away from my self. When I transfer over to the mode of inward-turned consciousness there arises an enlightened state of awareness concerning the nature of perception and the differences between self, mind, and body. The timeless and nonconceptual witnessing self is more readily felt as a *within* subjectivity. So now let me begin to seriously look within.

Let us cover two facets of this issue of sense perception and then summarize so that we may be brought back to the simple statement of point 2.3. The two facets of the sense perception issue can be stated thus:

1. By their very functioning, the sensory systems build illusory perceptions.
2. I falsely project my inner perceptions out into the external realities—as though the perceptions themselves *take place* in the external reality. In this way there arises an entire network of illusion about the self's relation to the external reality.

Now we can examine these two facets in greater detail.

How does self make contact with the external reality? The most immediate and obvious way is through the senses of the material body. Second by second I sensually investigate and interact with external reality, with the *out there*. This external reality, the out there, appears before me as a gigantic energy system in a continual state of flux—endless names, endless forms. This living waking dream is composed of sun and stars and moon, oceans and clouds, humans and animals and plants, meadows and mountains, movement and stillness, wetness and dryness, sounds and smells, heat and cold—unlimited things and unlimited relationships between things. Though I conceive of it all as being out there, certainly in a more valid sense my individual experience of out there takes place *within*. Whatever I pick up through my senses gets reconstructed within through my inner faculties, and thus my observations and my *reality*, though apparently external, are in fact self-constructed interior domains.

The eyes, ears, and tactile sense are the primary agents in the formation of my profane self—my *feeling* of physical being. It is through these sense organs, their perceptions, and my ideas about the nature of their perceptions that my rigid interlock with and bondage to the phenomenal exterior world takes place. Through the perceptions of these sense organs I feel a connection to and enslavement by the objects of sense perception. Most persons consider that their sense experience gives them an accurate, trustworthy, and complete perspective on reality. But by studying the mechanics of the sense-perceptual processes, we can understand that this sensory perspective is not only inaccurate and incomplete but also illusory. Again, though I seem to experience the external reality as if it is *out there,* for me the world is an illusory self-constructed interior domain.

The world of matter is inherently dark. I see by the aid of various localized luminaries. When there is no light I do not see the outside reality, because vision is dependent on light. Light must be reflected from an object in order for me to perceive that object. The reflected light leaves the *out there* and passes through the outer boundaries of the spherical globes of flesh known as the eyes. Under the influence of the eyes' lenses the light forms inverted images on the nerve-rich back wall of the eyes known as the retina. There the light causes chemical reactions. These reactions stimulate millions of specialized nerve cells that in turn produce trains of electrical impulses. These impulses quickly pass along the optic nerves until they reach the brain, the body's organ for arranging the chaotic arrays of sensory signals. There they are reconstructed from the electrical-impulse form into coded symbolic form.

Vedic authorities describe how, at this point, the subtle medium of mind takes over. It is the distinct element of mind, a subtle entity different from the brain, which makes a kind of sensory reality out of all these gross physical events. Mind is the link between the seeing mechanism and the seer (self). So when a tree appears before my eyes, there is an undeniable entity known as *tree* objectively speaking, but for me, the observer, there is nothing more than an internalized, limited, delayed reconstruction of a train of electrical impulses, which have been fed in to the brain along the pathway of the optic nerves. As seer I experience not the object but the symbolic reconstruction of the object within the brain through conscious interpretation by the mind. Though I mistakenly think that my seeing and reality somehow go on *out there,* in fact it is all an illusory and imperfectly constructed interior domain. Seeing and that which is seen are not outside; it is all an internal affair. When one has finally let go of the false identification with the psychosomatic structures the division between the so-called outside and inside will no longer be an issue.

The mechanics of my auditory perceptions carry the same illusory stigma as my visual perceptions. I consider that the sound vibrations (minute changes in air pressure caused by a vibrating object) are being perceived as if *out there,* when in fact, they are being composed within by the brain's reconstruction of nerve impulses leading this time from the ears and consequently interpreted by the mind. I project the perception *outward* to its vibrating source, though the actual perception takes place *within.* The mechanics of auditory perception are as gross and physical as the eyes' business of transforming patterns of light into nerve impulses. By the movements of membranes, rods, levers, liquids, and finally tiny receptor hair cells, there is the resultant train of auditory nerve impulses into the brain, along with their interpretation into meaningful patterns (in-formation). The sound is not really out there for the hearer, but rather it is within. My individual experiences of the barking dog, the ringing bell, or the sound of the closing door—though seeming to be external—are in fact illusory and imperfectly constructed interior domains of *sound*.

Though my senses of taste and smell contribute somewhat to my sense of physical being and feeling, it is the continuous sensation of touch that forms my final major perceptual interlock with the external world. This sensory system involves a number of tactile organs that register such diverse sensations as spatial awareness, heat, cold, pressure, wetness, and air movements. The essential mechanism of all these perceptions consists of sensory receptors situated under the skin throughout the entire body that respond to external stimuli from the environment. As before, the actual perceptions of the *out there* situation take place within the mind.

The immediate physical directness and pervasiveness of this continual assault of tactile sensory impressions (such as pressure, temperature, and humidity) very powerfully establish the illusion of outward bodily feeling and boundary. My sense of identity mixed with this array of outward-projected perceptions causes such feelings as "I am hot," "I am wet," or "I am cold," when in fact I am none of these perceptions. Though I feel and witness the heat, moisture, or absence of heat to be at the surface of the skin of the body, the truer reality of these perceptions exists not on the outward surface of the body but rather deeper within, closer to the self, in the subtle sheaths of mind energy.

Through these very brief descriptions of the physical actions of the sense organs of vision, hearing, and touch, it has been shown that the world, though objectively existing *out there,* is for me nothing more than an interpretation of incomplete and superficial sensory data received through an ingenious yet imperfect arrangement of bodily parts—organs whose designs necessarily create illusion. This imperfection is nicely summed up in the *Katha Upanishad,* fourth division, wherein it is stated:

The Creator made the senses outward-going: they go to the world of matter outside, not to the spirit within.

My senses are not instruments for knowledge. They are better designed for *avidya,* ignorance. The design of the material body is just right for ignorance and illusion, so that I can enact a role of false selfhood upon the relative plane. This sensory arrangement and its reactions push me strongly toward illusory conceptions of myself, the phenomenal manifestation surrounding me, and my relationship with that manifestation. The individual power of the separate organs to create illusory conceptions of reality through the mind is greatly multiplied when the input from the entire organism (all the perceptive senses) is being fed into the brain and interpreted by the mind all at the same time. Then I am bound up, as it were, by a continuous overlapping array of sensory stimuli with little hope of true perceptual clarity. But clarity is definitely possible through the combination of analytical understanding and actions performed on the soul platform—devotional service— especially the mode of devotional service recommended for this age, the chanting and hearing of the mahamantra.

In the Bhaktivedanta purports to the *Bhakti-rasamrta-sindhu,* or *The Nectar of Devotion,* chapter 3, it is pointed out that the analytical approach, *jnana,* must be mixed with the worship of the Godhead for one to have steadiness and permanence in the evolution of spiritual consciousness.

> Without being elevated to the position of a *jnani,* one cannot stick
> to the principle of worshipping the Supreme Personality of Godhead
> ... The *jnani* is one who has thoroughly understood that he is spirit
> soul and not simply a body.

Therefore, as I begin worshipping the Supreme Personality of Godhead through the sublime method of hearing and chanting the mahamantra, I will carefully try to understand my true identity as spirit soul and not the body. Once I have understood the basic mechanics of the sensory systems and know the illusion that they create, as well as how they create the illusion, then there is a loosening of the grip of illusion, and the false identification of self as body begins to fall away. When false ego is diminished, then the practice of mahamantra yoga becomes more and more effective.

I will alter the thinking processes to see that thoughts are carefully aimed at reducing rather than increasing the idealized self-image or ego. Physical sensations should be thought of in relation to the body and not to the self. Not "I am cold"; better to think, "my body is cold," or "there is a sensation of coldness occurring." Not "I am seeing"; think, "my body is seeing," or "seeing is occurring." Or better still, "In this wonderful way there are illusory visual impressions through the interactions of light, eyes, nerves, brain, mind, and self."

I graphically imagine being able to turn off the various senses one by one and then turn them on once again. With such ability there would be a marked shift in my attitude toward sense perception. I must break down all sensory experiences into their elemental components and divorce the conscious-observer principle (self) from such experiences. Then, before beginning to practice mahamantra yoga, consider the gateways between the conscious self and the external world. These gateways are the five sensory systems.

Point 2.4
Neglect the measuring and planning functions of the mind.

> uddhared atmanatmanam
> natmanam avasadayet
> atmaiva hy atmano bandhur
> atmaiva ripur atmanah

[Translation:]

A man must elevate himself by his own mind, not degrade himself.
The mind is the friend of the conditioned soul, and his enemy as well.

(*BHAGAVAD-GITA:* 6–5)

> *bandhur atmatmanas tasya*
> *yenatmaivatmana jitah*
> *anatmanas tu satrutve*
> *vartetatmaiva satruvat*

[Translation:]

For him who has conquered the mind, the mind is the best of friends, but for one who has failed to do so, his very mind will be the greatest enemy.

(*Bhagavad-gita:* 6–6)

The mind has a strong tendency in its "enemy" stage to *make plans* for its various sensory pursuits. It also possesses the parallel tendency to *measure* the bombardment of sense impressions from outside sources to determine just where, when, and how it may encounter either the greatest degree of gratification from those sources or the greatest circumstances for safety from those sources. In fact the material world and material consciousness is described by Vedic authorities as the realm of *kuntha*—the place possessed of the characteristic of measuring everything—as differing from the spiritual plane of *Vaikuntha,* which is devoid of all relative measuring and planning tendencies. These tendencies can arise prior to and during the practice of mahamantra yoga as thoughts such as, "When I finish this spiritual practice, I will go to the store." "As I chant with open eyes on my '*japa* walk,' the sunrise is very beautiful." "This man or this woman now passing before me is very attractive." "There are six rounds left until I finish my prescribed number of rounds of mahamantra meditation, so in some thirty to forty-five minutes I should be finished and will be able to do other things."

Much of the planning and measuring tendency in its grosser aspects can be avoided simply by moving the locus of awareness to the heart organ and closing the eyes. There is no need at all to open the eyes during the practice of mahamantra yoga. I can evolve the hearing function as though I were a blind person.

Before starting the practice of mahamantra yoga, I shall disregard all plans, all past and future, and all measurements of sensory data. I should transfer such tendencies to the counting beads that are used in the individual practice of mahamantra meditation. There is nothing to plan or measure; I have only to hear and chant the mahamantra and pull the counting beads when appropriate.

Point 2.5
Residing in the organ of the heart as atomic sentience, lucidly visualize entrance into the four profound inner states described in the third verse of Sri Chaitanya Mahaprabhu's Sri Sri Siksastaka.

This is the most important of all instructions on the hearing and chanting of the mahamantra. If I can concentrate on only one principle during my practice of mahamantra yoga, then let me concentrate on this principle.

> *trinad api sunichena*
> *taror iva sahishnuna*
> *amanina manadena*
> *kirtaniyah sada hari*

[Translation:]
> One can chant the Holy Name of the Lord in a humble state of mind, thinking oneself lower than the straw in the street, more tolerant than the tree, devoid of all sense of false prestige, and ready to offer all respects to others. In such a state of mind, one can chant the Holy Name of the Lord constantly.

The Supreme Lord Himself is giving within this instruction the key to the ceaseless chanting of the mahamantra. In this age my salvation from the dualistic relative plane of birth and death is through 100 percent association with the Supreme Pure in His sound-vibration incarnation. But in the beginning the materially contaminated mind has no taste for hearing and chanting, not to mention performing the activity ceaselessly. In his *Sri Upadesamrta*, text 7, Srila Rupa Goswami compares the materially conditioned state to the disease known as jaundice. When one has jaundice, the ayurvedic cure is to eat sugar candy. Even though it is a very sweet medicine, to the tongue of the diseased person the sugar candy tastes bitter. Nevertheless, if one tolerates the apparently bitter taste and continues to take the sugar candy, the disease eventually goes away. Then the intrinsic sweetness of the medicine is fully revealed. Similarly, if I will just go on with my hearing and chanting of the mahamantra in deep and abiding faith and concentration, in the *state of mind* indicated by Sri Chaitanya Mahaprabhu in His third verse of *Sri Sri Siksastaka* then the supremely blissful, eternal spiritual character of Sri Nama Avatara is revealed to me by Sri Nama Avatara Himself.

It's important to look closely at this third verse. I notice that the statement is not to chant humbly but rather to engage in the chanting in a humble *state of mind*. There is quite a difference between the two. I am seeking total states of mind here, not shallow sentimentality. What is it like to be lower than the straw in the street? Stated in the direct, visual language of the *Sri Sri Siksastaka,* it is to reduce the sense of identity to the atomic scale. I visualize a street from a new perspective, as a vast and gigantic stretch of flat surface many miles across. On this street I visualize a tiny piece of straw, appearing now as massive as some large mountain range. I am now lower than the straw in the street. How large does that make me? I feel profoundly just how tiny I really am—perhaps as small as the Upanishads' description of the self as "one ten-thousandth the tip of a hair." This state of mind is required.

But I am not in the human body any longer. I have now assumed the form of a tree. There is wind—I tolerate. There is snow and ice—I tolerate. There is tremendous heat—I tolerate. Someone has come to take my leaves and branches—I tolerate. I am fixed in my place and immovable. This state of mind is required.

My sense of identity has been reduced to its actual atomic size, so now I have no place in human society. I am too small to be noticed. I have no position among the men and women of the world. All sense of prestige is now gone from my life. This state of mind is required.

I am now like the minuscule tree, fixed and immovable, dwarfed by the vastness of the environment, with no place in human society. People step on me—I offer them my respects. Dogs step upon me—I offer them my respects. I am a resilient little tree, and I spring back each time with respect toward those who would love me or to those who would crush me. This state of mind is required.

My consciousness is transformed from its usual perspective of "five foot ten." I will assume my role as *atomic sentience* and practice it at all times. I will go on chanting the mahamantra and without a doubt He will inject me with spiritual energy and pure knowledge that enables me to act from the true perspective. When my chanting and hearing enter into union with the conceptions of this verse of the *Sri Sri Siksastaka,* then I experience unobstructed access to and strong desire for ceaseless chanting and hearing. Chanting becomes so sweet that I cannot stop. I chant on and on. This verse ushers me into the spiritual world. Through its intensive application in the practice of mahamantra yoga, I realize the spiritual nature of the mahamantra. I can finally understand that the mahamantra is not like the ordinary sounds of this material world. I now know that Sri Nama Avatara is immense—eternal—blissful. My attitude toward Him is far different from what it was before. My hairs stand on end; my eyes fill with tears; my voice chokes up. My faith in and love of the mahamantra deepens immensely, and I come to the realization that the mahamantra is absolute sound vibration—infinite Godhead as sound.

Point 2.6
Complete the mental foundations for mahamantra yoga by firmly fixing the locus of awareness in the heart and meditating upon the Sri panca-tattva mantra.

The Supreme Personality of Godhead's mercy is the key element in spiritual progress. Lord Sri Chaitanya Mahaprabhu and His associates have come in this dark age known as the Kali Yuga to give the mercy of hearing and chanting of the mahamantra. Only through Their favor can anything of a spiritual nature be accomplished without the great difficulty of previous ages and the methods then employed. The pure *vaisnavism* of Sri Chaitanya and His followers is known by some as "the science of mercy." Their beneficence can be predicted with accuracy. Meditate upon the panca-tattva mantra and I am blessed by Them with "the competency to chant the Hare Krishna mahamantra without offence" (Bhaktivedanta purports, *Sri Chaitanya-caritamrta, Adi-lila*, 7.168). Chant Their names and very soon the most exalted states of pure transcendental love of God are available for the sincere and earnest mahamantra yogis.

Sri Chaitanya Mahaprabhu and His associates are both the givers of the mahamantra and also the channel to the perfect chanting of the mahamantra. With great reverence, love, and attention I will always precede my practice of hearing and chanting the mahamantra with the chanting of the panca-tattva mantra:

> *sri-krishna-chaitanya prabhu nityananda*
> *sri-advaita gadadhara*
> *srivasadi-goura-bhakta-vrinda.*

Such chanting will always produce an auspicious outcome.

3 Production

The physical and mechanical aspects of chanting

Always chanting My glories, endeavoring with great determination, bowing down before Me, these great souls perpetually worship Me with devotion.

SRI KRISHNA *BHAGAVAD-GITA* 9:14

The short third chapter of this book takes up the production of the physical or outward manifestation of Sri Nama Avatara. The full manifestation of the unlimited glories of Sri Nama Avatara does not come about simply by an exertion of the various vocal organs. Any literate person can read aloud the mahamantra. But that does not mean that the reader is instantly in full realization of the Supreme Personality of Godhead. The completeness of the realization evolves along with the purity of the chanter. We will talk about the subtleties of these topics in greater detail in chapter 5. For now we will simply delve in to some of the mechanisms that go into the production of the outward manifestation of Sri Nama Avatara. The following thirty-two syllables compose the mahamantra (pronounced ha'- ray, krish'-na, and ra'-ma):

Hare Krishna Hare Krishna Krishna Krishna Hare Hare
Hare Rama Hare Rama Rama Rama Hare Hare.

Point 3.1
Produce the outward manifestation of Sri Nama Avatara by a vigorous coordinated effort of breath, vocal cords, jaw, tongue, and lips.

This is a simple and direct statement that can be understood by any study of the function of the vocal mechanism. Clear chanting of the mahamantra as well as clear speech requires the activation of all of these elements. Such activation must be vigorously undertaken. A lazy or slovenly approach will not be effective. This point is touched upon in the Bhaktivedanta purports of the *Sri Chaitanya-caritamrta, Adi-lila* 17.32, wherein it is mentioned:

> Chanting involves the activities of the upper and lower lips as well as the tongue. All three must be engaged in chanting the Hare Krishna mahamantra. The words "Hare Krishna" should be very distinctly pronounced.

In the beginning of my practice of mahamantra yoga I will pay attention to enunciate the mahamantra, then quickly it becomes second nature and the sound produced is at least phonetically accurate. This is the starting point in the actual practice of chanting and hearing the mahamantra.

Point 3.2
To sharpen enunciation of the mahamantra, silently ask "Who?"

This is a simple and sensible exercise that can help me to chant clearly. The question "Who?" strongly implies personality. Specific persons have specific names. The "who" I am referring to is the Supreme Personality of Godhead, Krishna. When I ask "Who?" I cannot help but say clearly the name, "Krishna." If I notice that my pronunciation of the mahamantra is becoming unclear, then, utilizing no more than a fraction of a second, I mentally consider the question "Who?"

Point 3.3
While chanting and hearing the mahamantra, let breathing take care of itself.

I will let the breathing take place in its natural unconscious way, just as I do during normal speaking. I will not worry about getting enough air to breathe but will simply let any awareness of breath fall away beneath my conscious awareness. Though I employed conscious breathing earlier to stabilize my mind and turn it inward, now I will drop the attention from breathing and focus upon the production, the enunciation, of the transcendental sound vibration.

Point 3.4
While chanting and hearing the mahamantra, let speed be subservient to clear hearing.

Here let me consider the adage "anything worth doing is worth doing well." There is no activity in my life more valuable than hearing and chanting the mahamantra. Though chanting too slowly is seldom a problem, in the beginning I may tend to chant too quickly. I will avoid chanting so quickly that I lose clarity. In ordinary life would I speak so quickly that no one could understand a word I was saying? What would be the value of such speaking?

A student being punished for some misdeed may be required to write some repetitive and (perhaps to the student) meaningless phrase on the blackboard. The student may consider the activity to be dull and useless and may try to repeat it very quickly to be finished with it. After a while the written words may become unintelligible both to the teacher and to the student. Is mahamantra yoga a dull and painfully repetitive activity or exercise? Am I to complete my numerical vow of chanting the mahamantra in the mood of this impatient student?

As I am moved over into the transcendental sphere of chanting I notice that Sri Nama Avatara Himself is the regulator of all aspects of the hearing and chanting endeavor. Sri Nama Avatara will speed up or slow down the chanting. I am not the controller of Sri Nama Avatara; rather Sri Nama Avatara controls me.

Point 3.5
While chanting and hearing the mahamantra let volume be subservient to clear hearing.

I shall chant loudly enough so that I can hear the sound. Murmuring—what His Divine Grace A. C. Bhaktivedanta Swami Prabhupada refers to as a "hissing sound"—is sometimes thought by neophytes to be the practice of mahamantra yoga. In fact though, this is not the practice of mahamantra yoga. I will find it much easier to fix my mind on the mahamantra when I chant at a moderate pace and volume.

Point 3.6
Let musical dimensions in mahamantra yoga play a minor, complimentary, nondistracting role and nothing more.

Here *kirtana*, the congregational chanting of the mahamantra, is being discussed. Naturally, congregational chanting means a degree of musical setting, with various melodies and instruments. The vibrations are on occasion very beautiful from the mundane musical perspective. Sometimes a materialist considers the kirtana quite beautiful and sometimes considers it nothing more than disturbing noise. I disregard all the relative material conceptions of "good" or "not so good" kirtana.

Let us recall the history of Srila Bhaktisiddhanta Saraswati Thakura, another of the great acaryas of mahamantra yoga, who would at times direct that the kirtana be chanted without any regard for the accepted standards of mundane musical performance. The pitch of the singer might be completely off. Or other more melodious kirtana singers would be bypassed by his request for those kirtana leaders of a higher degree of spiritual attainment and purity. The musical character of the kirtana was not given very much importance; rather it was eclipsed by the substance of the higher conceptions.

The quality of the kirtana depends on the chanters' pure conception of the mahamantra, on their absorption in the mahamantra, and on their realizations while chanting the mahamantra. I need not overly concern myself with musical details. A kirtana having lovely musical characteristics but lacking absorption of the mind or purity of conception is soon forgotten. "Just another kirtana." When a kirtana has modest musical characteristics but the chanters have the pure conception, full absorption, and ever-increasing transcendental consciousness—then the kirtana will never be forgotten.

Whatever musical instruments I use to accompany the kirtana should complement my fundamental purpose of intensified hearing and chanting of the mahamantra. The instruments should not direct my mind to themselves but to the mahamantra. The melody should not direct my mind to itself but to the mahamantra. A sweet, sentimental melody is not necessarily the best. Fancy or excessively loud *mrdunga* drum playing is not necessarily the best. Giant crashing kartalas are not necessarily the best. If my attention is to something other than the mahamantra during the kirtana, then I have missed the essential point of chanting. The Lord is pleased by higher and higher manifestations of spiritual love, not by the dexterity of the harmonium player or the vibrato of the various chanters. The superior kirtana may be during a very simple gathering where only the hands are being clapped. I will strive for purity. I will not try to force ecstasy by the beat of the drum. I must first chant and hear and then know definitely that all wonderful qualities will follow. As soon as I neglect to approach the mahamantra as transcendental sound vibration and begin to give stress to the musical details, at that time I begin my journey away from the true path of mahamantra yoga and I enter upon the pitted road of dissatisfaction of the heart.

4 Identification

Explaining the realities of the
mahamantra to the mind

*There are specific modes of perception, which help in our
efforts to grasp the infinite.*

GOETHE

This fourth chapter talks about conceptions of Sri Nama Avatara that
we should evoke during our hearing and chanting of the mahamantra.
Our theme and title comes from the expression "explain to the mind"
found in Srila Bhaktivinoda Thakura's 1893 essay "Nama-bhajana."

In its conditioned state the mind will hinder our progress. It will try
to make everything material. Even though Sri Nama Avatara is supremely
spiritual the material mind will attempt to reduce the transcendental
sound vibration to the status of mere "songs" or "auspicious chants" or
"Indian folk observances." The mahamantra has no such relative limita-
tion. This chapter will help us to overcome this tendency of placing material conceptions upon the transcendental reality of Sri Nama Avatara.

We must contend with still another limiting feature of the mind.

40

Generally mind cannot clearly hold more than one thought or focus at a time. Our awareness of one thought makes it impossible to be simultaneously aware of other thoughts. Now, the points of this very chapter comprise many thoughts. So how are we to remain aware of these many other thoughts at the time of trying to hear and chant the mahamantra?

To answer this question let us remember ideas that were mentioned in the introduction. This book has been arranged in a way that may be easily understood by the analytical mind. The entire presentation has been divided into chapters, and the chapters have been divided into points. The order that has been utilized is reasonable and sensible. This order has been so devised to facilitate the acquisition of the various conceptions of this book. But, once hearing and chanting the mahamantra has started, there is not necessarily any fixed order of events. Points that are found in chapter 5 might become prominent within the mind before some of the points mentioned in chapter 4.

So we should concentrate foremost upon hearing in our practice of mahamantra yoga. In the early stages the mind's ability to focus without distraction will be broken repeatedly. The points of this book dealing with the higher conceptions of Sri Nama are to be injected at those times of broken attention. We then refocus our attention upon the transcendental sound vibration. Hear, inject the higher conceptions, hear, inject the higher conceptions, and so on. Once we surpass this mechanical stage by entering within the internal forest, the plane of transcendence, then Sri Nama Avatara Himself intervenes on our behalf and we do not have to concern ourselves with the mechanical process of focusing the mind. Then we will be in the camp of the true forest dwellers, the *vanavasis*.

In this chapter we will discuss eight points that will counteract these tendencies of the conditioned mind.

Point 4.1
Know Sri Nama Avatara to be the Supreme Person, the dynamic and vital Godhead, who directly acts within our life's course.

Sri Nama Avatara comes to me as sound. In my life's experience I know spoken sounds to be nothing more than verbal utterances possessing mutually agreed upon meanings that are different from *the thing itself.* The sound is not the thing represented. The sound is different from the object. The mahamantra is not that kind of relative sound vibration.

When an entity has a form that I can experience, then I can easily attribute personal characteristics to the entity. For instance, my experience in worshiping the divine forms of the Lord in the temple, the *arca-murti,* has proved that form establishes a sense of personality. In time I will also begin to recognize the extremely personal *form* of Sri Nama Avatara, the absolute sound form that is just as personal as the arca-murti, the Deity in the temple. The sound form known as Sri Nama Avatara is supremely personal.

Two human beings can talk to each other, express certain feelings, and exhibit various characteristics. Though to my conditioned mind the mahamantra may seem an abstract entity, He relates to me in the most personal manner imaginable. Because Sri Nama Avatara knows my innermost thoughts and desires, He is able to relate to me in profoundest intimacy. He reciprocates with me, and I can note this exchange time after time. The give-and-take exchanges can be very pronounced and are primarily based upon my faith in Sri Nama Avatara. There is no question of Sri Nama Avatara having faith in my existence. He is the Absolute Cognizance. He is fully aware of my existence. When I expand and purify my faith in Sri Nama Avatara and His supreme existence, then there is greater and greater scope for reciprocation. Exchange of love requires two persons who believe in one another. I believe deeply in the personal reality of the mahamantra, and wonderful exchanges of love with Sri Nama Avatara are mine to cherish.

My deep faith in Sri Nama Avatara will uncover the reality of His dynamic nature, and I will see Him as the loving and kind master who gives direction and guidance. *I will clearly perceive and feel the direct intervention that Sri Nama Avatara exerts within my life.* His actions and involvement within my life will become very clear. He moves me. He enlightens me.

Point 4.2

Know Sri Nama Avatara to be eternally spiritual—above material phenomena and distinct from all other sound vibrations.

Sri Nama Avatara descends into the material world to help everyone. Though He appears to be in the time and space dimensions of the relative plane, He is untouched by matter. He exists on the eternal plane of bliss and knowledge. In the beginning I accept, at least theoretically, point 4.2 and build my faith from there. Sri Nama Avatara is absolute sound vibration.

Sri Nama Avatara reveals His spiritual nature to the sincere and faithful candidate. The process spirals deeply into an ever-increasing revelation. First, proportionate to my faith in Sri Nama Avatara, Sri Nama Avatara will reciprocate by revealing something of His spiritual nature to me. As my faith deepens, Sri Nama Avatara will reveal more to me. As a result my faith will deepen further, and greater and greater revelations will take place. One day I will feel very sorry that I could ever have considered the mahamantra to be anything like ordinary sound. One day I will wake up from the dream. Past conceptions of the mahamantra will be blown away like specks of dust in a great gale, and I will see the eternal form clearly before me. Sri Nama Avatara then will appear to me as the limitless and loving controller, the Supreme Person who exists in eternity.

Point 4.3

Know Sri Nama Avatara as the primary reality in the super-excellent spiritual process for expansion of personal consciousness and realization of the ultimate truths of existence.

The process of bhakti-yoga is the natural and eloquent process of spiritual advancement for the conditioned living entities in the material world. This statement is not the by-product of a sectarian dualistic thought process. The thread of bhakti—purified unmotivated devotion of the eternal spiritual self to the supreme Self—runs through every major spiritual path that humanity has ever known. It is so strong that it even develops within nontheistic schools such as Buddhism. The tendency to serve and devote oneself to some higher cause abounds. It filters outward from the soul platform through the various layers of matter into our immediate material experience as the "isms" such as socialism, communism, humanitarianism, and nationalism.

Devotional service is the eternal characteristic of all living beings. As sugar always gives sweetness, so the soul always gives service. Service cannot be separated from the self, and it does not stop. When this characteristic is purified and brought into relationship with the Supreme Personality of Godhead, then it is known by the name bhakti-yoga. A candid and unbiased comparison of bhakti with various other paths will show the fruits of many of these other paths to be wonderful, though perhaps not final. The mahamantra yogis suggest that the fruits of all spiritual paths are eventually revealed to be tributaries leading to the vast raging river of bhakti. It is not the purpose of this book to go into detail about the nature of bhakti and its relation to the various paths available to the human species. The reader may refer to the devotional books listed in the bibliography to get a detailed account of the path of bhakti-yoga. Here we should simply note that on the path of bhakti, the essential ingredient for advancement in this current age, Kali Yuga, is contact with the transcendental sound of Sri Nama Avatara through the mercy of His pure devotees.

Nevertheless, within the teachings of Sri Chaitanya Mahaprabhu we are brought to a perspective where we may consider the possibilities that bhakti just might take the astanga-yogis beyond the various levels of samadhi, that it could perhaps transport the jnanis far past the nondifferentiated oneness of the eternality of the brahmic splendor, and that the various perfections of divine emptiness as found in schools of Eastern and Western Gnosticism might be conceived and perceived by the perfected mahamantra-yogis as but different perspective views of the brahmic splendor and thus are considered to be like way stations on the astounding journey toward the super-excellent realization of the Lord's abode, Goloka Vrindavana. And hazy conceptions of "heaven" or "paradise" of theistic traditions such as Christianity, Islam, or Judaism could perhaps be brought into a focus of crystal clarity through the science of bhakti-yoga. In the bhakti tradition one realizes the extensive and astounding details.

Much of humanity's documented mystical experience concerns the realization of *sat*, the Godhead's aspect of eternity. But simple eternality is not all in all, just as waking up in a dark room is not the complete expression of wakefulness. There is more, much more. Might we not then seek the Godhead's aspect of *ananda*, or infinite blissfulness through loving reciprocation with Him in devotional service—our eternal function?

The need we feel to transform our ordinary consciousness to a higher state is evident from countless current and historical examples. Human beings are seldom content with the limited scope of everyday consciousness. Those with restraining or destructive tendencies (*tama-guna*) and with activating or chaotic tendencies (*raja-guna*) may pursue this felt need to transform ordinary consciousness through such practices as drug taking, ghost worship, and occultism.

Those of a more introspective, illuminating, or godly nature *sattva-guna* will seek other methods of consciousness expansion that elevate, that reawaken the soul's loving relationship with the supreme Soul. The oldest and most comprehensive written expression of this science of primordial consciousness appears in India's Vedic literature. Therein it is often stated that for this age the recommended way to transform profane consciousness to God consciousness is to hear and chant the mahamantra. As we learn from the *Brhat-naradiya Purana:*

> *harer nama harer nama harer namaiva kevalam*
> *kalau nasty eva nasty eva nasty eva gatir anyatha.*

[Translation:]

In this age of Kali there is no alternative, there is no alternative, there is no alternative for spiritual progress than to chant the holy name, chant the holy name, chant the holy name of the Lord.

When one has the good fortune to receive the chanting of the mahamantra from a bona fide acarya of mahamantra yoga, then the transformations of consciousness brought about by such chanting eventually become complete and final.

Point 4.4
Know that the mahamantra is far more than His ephemeral shadow manifestation, which sincere neophyte practitioners usually experience. The real Sri Nama Avatara, the full manifestation of Godhead, is not invoked by a mere exercise of one's vocal mechanism. Rather, He descends through the agency of His pure devotees from the inconceivable plane of Goloka Vrindavana.

The chanting of the pure devotee of Sri Nama Avatara and the chanting of the beginner are very different manifestations. To the inexperienced observer, the sounds may seem identical, but there is a great difference.

When the neophyte practitioner chants he injects many material conceptions into the sound. Having never experienced even a partial manifestation of the Godhead as divine sound vibration, he has a faith that is very shallow. His knowledge and understanding are incomplete. Such a neophyte's consciousness is enveloped by the material atmosphere. His immediate understanding of self is more closely linked to the body than to the soul. His hearing of the mahamantra is little different from his hearing of ordinary speech, and in actuality, he makes only slight distinction between the two. His approach to the mahamantra is external—he approaches from the outside. He looks at the mahamantra just as a child might look at some sophisticated piece of scientific equipment. What he sees is vague and nebulous, though it may possess unknown powers.

The pure devotee has a vastly different attitude and orientation toward the mahamantra. His conceptions have nothing to do with the material mind. The pure devotee of Sri Nama Avatara has realizations, not mere material conceptions, as the basis of his understanding. His faith is profound and powerful, for he knows with absolute certainty that Sri Nama Avatara is the eternal reality, the cause of all causes. The consciousness of the pure devotee exists within the spiritual atmosphere, while his material body appears before us within the material dimensions of time and space. Even though his material body is now spiritualized through incessant practice of bhakti-yoga he has fully realized that his identity is utterly different from that body. The pure devotee also sees a clear distinction between material sound vibrations and the pure spiritual sounds that have direct relation to the Supreme Personality of Godhead. He does not look at the mahamantra from the outside and at a distance but rather he lives in the mahamantra, and he communes with Sri Nama Avatara in purest atemporal love.

The true mahamantra flows from the Goloka Vrindavana plane into the material world through the mouths of His pure devotees. I should, if at all possible, receive the mahamantra from such pure realized souls, because only they can deliver the full manifestation of Sri Nama Avatara. Those less pure will give me something less—an offense to Sri Nama Avatara or a dim reflection of Sri Nama Avatara. Because pure devotees of Sri Nama Avatara are very rare within human society, I should consider myself extremely fortunate to contact them. My sincere dedication to the goals of mahamantra yoga is my only hope for somehow receiving the causeless mercy of Sri Nama Avatara's pure devotee. Once having made contact with the pure devotee, I will adopt the mood of his menial servant, ask him appropriate questions about spiritual advancement, and hear from him about such topics as confirmed in the *Bhagavad-gita* 4.34:

> *tad viddhi pranipatena*
> *pariprasnena sevaya*
> *upadeksyanti te jnanam*
> *jnaninas tattva-darsinah*

[Translation:]

> Just try to learn the truth by approaching a spiritual master. Inquire from him submissively and render service unto him. The self-realized souls can impart knowledge unto you because they have seen the truth.

When I serve the completely pure devotees of Sri Nama Avatara, I begin to acquire their transcendental qualities and so become fit to receive the transcendental sound vibration. This point is nicely made in the *Srimad-Bhagavatam* 1:2–16, wherein it is stated:

> O twice-born sages, by serving those devotees who are completely freed from all vice, great service is done. By such service, one gains affinity for hearing the messages of Vasudeva (Krishna).

This eagerness to hear the transcendental sound vibration is one of the most important qualifications for advancement in the culture of mahamantra yoga.

But Sri Nama Avatara is not perceivable by the material senses. The simple movements of the tiny membranes of skin known as the eardrums do not qualify me to receive Sri Nama Avatara. Being transcendental, Sri Nama Avatara is beyond the ken of any material perceptual instrument. He exists beyond the minute changes in air pressure produced by the vibrating straps of flesh within the throat. His presence and reality do not depend on any mechanical device that might seem needed to *produce* Him. Break down the material medium, remove the air molecules, and Sri Nama Avatara will continue to exist—just as He always has and always will. The *Padma Purana* sums up the entire point in the verse:

> *atah sri-Krishna namadi na bhaved grahyam indriyaih*
> *sevonmukhe hi jivadau svayam eva sphuraty adah*

[Translation:]

> No one can understand the transcendental nature of the name, form, quality, and pastimes of Sri Krishna through his materially contaminated senses. Only when one becomes spiritually saturated by transcendental service to the Lord are the transcendental name, form, quality, and pastimes of the Lord revealed to him.

Point 4.5

Know that Sri Nama Avatara is the gatekeeper—the resplendent regulator—of the expansion and contraction of one's personal consciousness.

Point 4.5 will become very clear as soon as I enter upon the transcendental plane. At that time I will know that Sri Nama Avatara controls the entire spectrum of elements that make up my existence; from my physical body's movements, to my mind's thinking processes, to the very character of my consciousness. In a split second Sri Nama Avatara can open my consciousness and reveal an unobstructed view of the spiritual plane, and in the same small span of time close such a vision. Just as in the *Bhagavad-gita* when Lord Krishna astonishes his disciple Arjuna through the revelation of His *visva-rupa,* or "universal form," saying, *pasya me partha rupani*—"Behold my universal form!"—so Sri Nama Avatara can impress upon the tiny chanters His divine and astounding presence. I will be aware of the power and influence of the mahamantra within my life, and I will develop full dependence upon Him to awaken me from the dualistic confusion of material consciousness.

Point 4.6

Know that Sri Nama Avatara is the stupendously powerful agent who is ever eager to reveal, to those who love Him, limitless spiritual dimensions.

Sri Nama Avatara does not just reveal some partial level of transcendental awareness to His devotees; He opens up the limitless vista of the Goloka Vrindavana planet to that soul who has taken complete shelter in Him. A best friend will always invite you to his home.

Srila B. R. Sridhara Maharaja very beautifully elaborates upon this point in his book *The Search for Sri Krishna: Reality the Beautiful.* In chapter 12 he states:

So many charming aspects are shown as if to my eyes within, and He [Sri Nama Avatara] forcibly takes me to surrender at the foot of that altar. He shows Himself in His full-fledged form, in Vrindavana, in His *braja-lila,* with Radharani, and He takes me there. I find that I am in the midst of His peculiar, very sweet and loving paraphernalia. And He says, "You see! I have so many wonderful things. This is your home. I am not merely imagination, but concrete reality. You will find here that the environment is very favorable and sweet. You are to live here."

I believe deeply in the limitless wonder and power that abides within the mahamantra. I inject that faith and its conception into my practice of hearing and chanting. I will go on with it persistently, and one day my spiritual eyes will see everything. This awakening will definitely take place.

Point 4.7
Know that the activity of hearing and chanting the mahamantra is our plea for engagement in spiritual service at the divine lotus feet of Sri Sri Radha Krishna, Who are the same as Sri Nama Avatara.

There is no difference between the name of God and God Himself. The mahamantra is composed of three transcendental names: Hare, Krishna, and Rama. The meanings of these names is given in various places by various authorities. In the book *Teachings of Lord Kapila,* His Divine Grace A. C. Bhaktivedanta Swami Prabhupada clearly defines the meaning of "Hare." Therein he states:

> When we are chanting the mahamantra, we are actually making address to God and His energy Hara [Hare in the vocative]. Hara is Krishna's internal potency, Srimati Radharani. Thus the *Vaisnavas* worship *Radha-Krishna, Laksmi-Narayana,* and *Sita-Rama.* In the beginning of the Hare Krishna mahamantra we first address the internal energy of Krishna, Hare. Thus we say, "O Radharani! O Hare! O energy of the Lord!"

In the Bhaktivedanta purports to the *Srimad-Bhagavatam* 10.2, 11–12, it is further mentioned:

Vaisnavas are *suddha-saktas,* or pure *bhaktas,* because the Hare Krishna mahamantra indicates worship of the Supreme Lord's energy, *Hara.* A *Vaisnava* prays to the energy of the Lord for the opportunity to serve the Lord along with His spiritual energy.

The etymology of the name "Krishna" is found in the *Mahabharata Udyoga-parva,* 71.4, which says:

The word *krs* is the attractive feature of the Lord's existence, and *na* means spiritual pleasure. When the verb *krs* is added to the affix *na* it becomes *Krishna,* which indicates the Absolute Truth.

This explanation, along with many others, gives a clear meaning of this sweetest of names. The most simple and concise definition generally given is "the all-attractive Supreme Person." The name "Rama" is understood to mean "unlimited enjoyment of spiritual existence," which is none other than the Primeval Lord Himself in one of His most sublime aspects.

Shrivatsa Goswami in his interview with Steven J. Gelberg, found in the book *Hare Krishna, Hare Krishna: Five Distinguished Scholars on the Krishna Movement in the West,* gives a clear analysis of the grammatical character, construction, and meaning of the mahamantra. When asked about the meaning of the mantra and the identity of the sound "Hare" as "Radha" and "Rama" as "Krishna," Shrivatsa Goswami explains:

This is the seventh case ending, what you call in English the "vocative case"—when you are addressing or calling someone. In Sanskrit this is called *sambodhana,* "addressing." "Hare" is the vocative form of Hara. *Harati Krishna pranan iti hara:* "The one who attracts the whole being of Krishna is Hara." And that Hara is no other than Radha. When Radha is away from Krishna, Krishna is almost without life. That is the etymological meaning of Hara. "Radha" becomes "Radhe" and "Hara" becomes "Hare" in the vocative case. "Krishna" remains as "Krishna." So the mahamantra says, "Oh Radhe, Oh Krishna." And then "Krishna Krishna, Radhe Radhe." Each word in the mantra has this vocative ending.

In the second line, the new word is "Rama." *Ramayat redhikaya sa iti ramah:* "The one who sports with Radha is Rama." This "Rama" is Krishna. This is the meaning given by Jiva Goswami.

This mantra is so powerful because it is all in the form of a prayerful address. In other mantras you do not find this form of direct address. But in this mantra, each word is an address. Being in the form of an address, the force of the mantra is maximized . . . There cannot be a more forceful way to calling a name than in the direct address form. In the mahamantra, the prayer is focused on Krishna, and because it is focused, He is bound in that prayer.

A limitless realm of *rasa* (spiritually ecstatic taste) exists within the sound vibration of the mahamantra. Some of the wonders of that glorious plane of pleasure are exhibited as the eternal pastimes of Srimati Radharani and Lord Sri Krishna. I will regularly read about those pastimes from authoritative books such as *Srimad-Bhagavatam* and *Sri Brahma-samhita* and hear the proper explanation from the pure devotees of God. I will never divorce the beauty of those pastimes from the chanting and hearing of the mahamantra; rather, I will understand that there is eternal and absolute connection between what might appear as utterly unrelated features of the Personality of Godhead. The practice of mahamantra yoga is not merely some dry meditative process. It is much, much more. One day the greatest treasure of the mahamantra will be revealed to me, and gradually I will witness the disclosure of not only the name of the Godhead but also an awakening of awareness of the qualities, form, and pastimes of the Supreme Person as well.

Point 4.8

Know that by our hearing and chanting the mahamantra from the heart, we invoke the presence of our supreme, intimate Friend—our Shelter, Benefactor, Director, Lord, and Purifier—Who appears before us as the incarnation of divine sound.

This process of hearing and chanting the transcendental names of the Godhead is so very simple. Unfortunately, sometimes we feel that only through complicated, elaborate, and sophisticated arrangements are we able to do justice to our complicated egos. For us at those times, this process of chanting the mahamantra may seem too simple to be recognized for what it really is. We cannot see just how accessible and sublime this method of spiritual realization is for humankind.

If I have simple, uncomplicated faith, the mahamantra will take me very far. The mind cannot take me as far. My imagination stops short. I cannot imagine just how far Sri Nama Avatara can take me, since the planes and dimensions of that transcendental realm are totally beyond my experience—beyond my most vivid imaginings. The authoritative descriptions of the spiritual world exceed my capacity for comprehension. I will just try to have a little faith in Sri Nama Avatara and then scientifically test the process and experience the results. I will never be disappointed. As Lord Sri Krishna requests in *Brahma-samhita* 5.61:

Abandoning all meritorious performances serve Me with faith. The realization will correspond to the nature of one's faith.

And as we learn there in the purport given by the *acarya*, "The more transparent the faith, the greater the degree of realization."

हरे कृष्ण हरे कृष्ण

5 *Intensification*

The heightened focusing of mind when
Sri Nama Avatara begins to appear
within the chanter's ardent call

*The ideas which are here expressed so laboriously are
extremely simple and should be obvious. The difficulty lies
not in the new ideas, but in escaping from the old ones,
which ramify, for those brought up as most of us have been,
into every corner of our minds.*

JOHN MAYNARD KEYNES

This chapter describes the beginnings of actual transcendental realizations and our attitude toward those realizations. When Sri Nama Avatara begins to break into manifestation within our life, then we can know that our consciousness has undergone significant purification and is no longer entirely under the relative limitations of matter. Sri Nama Avatara does not appear within material consciousness.

This purification is not necessarily a long drawn-out affair, because Sri Nama Avatara can purify me within seconds if He so desires. When

I enter the reality of the internal forest and begin to directly experience Sri Nama Avatara, I will yearn to project myself deeper and deeper into that reality. The points in this chapter will act as catalysts to propel me into those wondrous depths. By that time I will have become one of "the living." I will perceive Sri Nama Avatara as an infinite personal being. My hearing and chanting of the mahamantra will have life. There will be cause both for celebration and for caution.

There are two divisions to this subject of intensification, one positive and one negative. In each the points are meant to assist in the practice of mahamantra yoga once the material body is transcended. The elaboration upon these points will be more of a technical or practical character rather than subjective or experiential. The descriptions of some of the internal realms that are obtainable through the practice of mahamantra yoga are given in chapter 6.

Part 1. Inclusive Approach to Intensification

Point 5.1
Now bring internal intensity to the foreground of consciousness.

The word "now" directs me to the idea of entrance into the transcendence. At this point in my practice I am leaving the material plane and emerging within the spiritual atmosphere. Though my physical body may be seated or standing in some particular time-and-space situation, my consciousness is not in that situation. My consciousness is "elsewhere." I find myself suddenly, mysteriously, within the realm of *sat*—eternity. My mouth continues chanting the mahamantra and my ears continue hearing the mahamantra, but Sri Nama Avatara, not my material ego, is in control. I know that I am very tiny, safe, and secure.

The words "internal intensity" imply that the total spectrum of elements that make up the inner person be directed utterly to the transcendental sound vibration. Sri Nama Avatara clearly helps me as I express my mood of reciprocation to have Him. He gives me what is necessary to have Him. Sri Nama Avatara makes me a true yogi though I feel that I have no material qualification. The stage of one-pointed-ness of mind, *ekagrata,* is readily obtained and then surpassed by the mercy of Sri Nama Avatara. Once contacted, Sri Nama Avatara makes it impossible for anything else to enter the mind. By my sincerity to be with Sri Nama Avatara, He brings Himself totally to the foreground of my being and awareness.

In his talk of September 18, 1931, to Dr. Magnus Hirschfield of Berlin, Srila Bhaktisiddhanta Saraswati Thakura described some of the characteristics of the transcendental sound vibrations of Sri Nama Avatara, as well as the concept of internal intensity.

The transcendental Sound has got distinctive character. The sound from the fourth dimension received by the ear has got a special potency to clear out all restricted ideas and to include everything of phenomena. The sounds we hear are meant to be restricted to the third dimension, to be transcended by the fourth and higher dimensions. The transcendental Sound clears out all impediments that block the path of the Sound.

The idea of immanence cannot be secured unless we break down the molecules. Unless we break them we cannot go to the other side and transcend time and space. That Sound will give a clear signal, a free path, by which we can make some progress toward the Absolute. That Sound should be received through instruction. We should undo what we have received hitherto. There will be no loss. The distinctive feature of that Sound is that it should incorporate all reciprocal objects along with the Sound. That Sound should not be neglected because of its distinctive quality as coming from the Transcendent and so includes all and at the same time comes with all potencies to clear out all sorts of un-aesthetic and wrong impressions received from our aptitude to enjoy the world, which should not hamper our progress toward the Full and Eternal.

We are only showing our natural aptitude and should not be denied. We should lend our ear to receive the transcendental Sound.

We should stop all our senses for the time being and receive the things and not merely the attributions. The transcendental Sounds are given us by the Fountainhead Who can take the initiative. He is not "It." He is to be deemed as Male-Moiety of the things of the subservient phenomena. The transcendental Sound should not lack any part of the Integer.

The transcendental Sound is equipped with All-potency. As the potency of Sound is restricted we find diverse existences in different things and are not in a position to receive things in full. Partial conceptions also make us forget. We should shake off all other ideas and thoughts for the time being. We expect the Absolute Language flowing into the ear to include all languages. If we behave otherwise, that Sound cannot communicate itself to us.

The transcendental Sound has got innumerable potencies. It has power of delegating power to us to receive all of it. When it comes from an unknown region it should first inject such power to our feeble receiving instrument as would enable us to welcome it. We must not show a challenging or rejecting attitude, as we are liable to do toward advice offered gratis.

We should know that the transcendental Sound has the necessary potencies that confer on us such desirable gifts as will enable us to neglect the other senses. Our eyes, nose, and so forth will be regulated by that Sound. This is not hypnotism or mesmerism that gives anthropomorphic ideas. The transcendental Sound will carry all the requisites necessary for receiving the sound. If we are desirous of catching the transcendental Sound we should be prepared for the time being to suspend all sensuous activities and wait for the transcendental Sound to include all.

Point 5.2
Direct the mind's focus to the aural field.

When Sri Nama Avatara begins to give access to His transcendental nature I will then focus my hearing even more intensely upon Him. I move in close to the sound vibrations and let my total being float within the presence of the Supreme Personality of Godhead. By the time this stage of hearing and chanting is reached, there are definite alterations of my conceptions and perceptions of self, spiritual existence, and body/mind/self relationships. I find that I cannot get too involved with any of the shifts in perception and ontology. I simply focus intensely on the ever-sweetening sound of the mahamantra.

Point 5.3
Garland the mind with the third verse of Sri Chaitanya Mahaprabhu's Sri Sri Siksastaka and vividly feel the four states again and again.

> One can chant the Holy Name of the Lord in a humble state of mind, thinking oneself lower than the straw in the street, more tolerant than the tree, devoid of all sense of false prestige, and ready to offer all respects to others. In such a state of mind one can chant the Holy Name of the Lord constantly.

It is my desire at this time of realization to nourish my adoration of Sri Nama Avatara. This verse of *Sri Sri Siksastaka* shall be the food. The mood and the states of mind offered by this beautiful verse of Sri Chaitanya Mahaprabhu will sustain my relationship with the living Godhead. The sweet and true environment of this verse will take me further and further. I feel the presence of Sri Chaitanya Mahaprabhu in His very words, and I try to capture the mood of His disposition and the vein of His goals. He is the Supreme Personality of Godhead, and He takes me to Himself, through Himself, as the transcendental sound vibration. His beautiful eternal golden dancing form of bliss now appears easily within the inner vision of my mind and He helps me to enter deeper and deeper into the wonders of the mahamantra without a doubt.

Earlier, in a devotionally mechanical way, I used the deeper meaning of this verse to bring me to the transcendental plane. Once material time and space are transcended, this verse enables me to remain transcendentally situated. Now mercy, not internal adjustments, is realized to be the dynamic factor bringing about my ultimate good.

Point 5.4
As a baby cries for its mother, move consciousnesses to the heart and cry for the shelter of Sri Nama Avatara.

This point does not simply act as analogy, it is the reality. This point offers a mood that can be employed throughout my culture of mahamantra yoga and now, at this dynamic starting point in my culture, it takes on a fantastic depth of sincerity. This atmosphere of utter dependence evolves and expands to invite envelopment by the comprehensive cloud of security. As I enter the internal forest of the heart by profound hearing and chanting of the mahamantra, I realize the cause of my very existence. The nature of that cause surprises me and amazes me, for truth is never as one imagines. Truth is beyond imagination.

Tiny children and babies cry when away from their parents. They have no shelter in the outer world. By crying they attract the shelter that they seek. I, as atomic sentience, am very, very tiny. I exist at the extreme end of the scale of sizes. The living entity is the infinitesimal—the smallest conscious fragment of existence—whereas the transcendental sound vibration of Sri Nama Avatara is the absolute infinitude. I have wandered away from my spiritual parents. I find myself adrift within a dark maze. Now my parents are near, manifesting before me as sound. They come close to me as I cry. The absolute personalities of Hare Krishna (or Radha Krishna) are the existential parents of all living beings. They have been waiting patiently to hear my call, and They eagerly come to pick me up.

For a long time I have been enveloped by the womb of the dense material energy and have been totally helpless and fearful. As soon as Sri Nama Avatara exerts His influence within the immediate environment, then I feel the shelter and safety of that situation. I am enveloped by a new kind of womb.

In the very beginning of my practice of mahamantra yoga, on occasion I felt blessed to be held by the embrace of Sri Nama Avatara. My life has been changed dramatically from that time onward. Having had this experience of profound security, I silently long to again be enveloped by the reality of the transcendental sound vibration. Let me build a great construction of desire for this state of being wrapped in the embrace of Sri Nama Avatara.

Point 5.5
As one standing helplessly on death's threshold, continue to practice mahamantra yoga in a noncontrolling mood.

The word "as" has been used and seems to point to analogy. However this is no more an analogy than point 5.4. This physical body *is* on death's threshold at every second. Only blind fools drowning in ignorance think otherwise. Before Sri Nama Avatara came into my life, before having met with the transcendental system of *guru-parampara,* I was held tightly within the grip of the destructible body. Though nearly always in utter denial of their impending death, great men and women of history, one by one, are crushed by it, and in the end all material persons go down to doom. Though I may enter the arena of life as a brave soldier about to conquer the world, in the end, unless I awaken spiritually, I die like a tiny bug under the intense heat of the desert sun.

Point 5.5 assists me in deepening and refining the preceding two points of practice and may also be utilized earlier in my practice as well. At this stage, as I make entrance into the realities of Sri Nama Avatara, I know that I am beyond death. Still I can understand that I am encased within a material body composed of hungry sense organs and could, without the protection of Sri Nama Avatara, fall easily from my newly acquired position. A child who has cried and just acquired the shelter of his parent's loving embrace does not push away from that embrace. The little child holds on tightly.

I will hold on tightly to Sri Nama Avatara by surrendering my false sense of control. I must feel as helpless as one who is suddenly faced with death. At an unannounced time when death unexpectedly greets me, no amount of material controlling egoism can help or change death's mind. I then must abandon my thinking as "controller" or "lord" and accept that I am the insignificant "controlled." And over the course of my life, haven't I seen this very thing in the eyes of so many living creatures as they enter into the gaping jaws of their demise? I have placed myself within the jaws of death and now cry out pitifully to Sri Nama Avatara for salvation.

Point 5.6
Feel strong love for Sri Nama Avatara—your savior.

I am not embarrassed or hesitant to love Sri Nama Avatara. I declare it boldly within my heart, and I strive to always think lovingly toward Him. Such thoughts will bear fruit just as in an arranged marriage the newly married young woman develops love for her husband by practicing thoughts of love toward him. In his small book, *The Bhagavata: Its Philosophy, Its Ethics, and Its Theology,* Srila Bhaktivinoda Thakura summarizes this point in the following statement: "No thought is useless. Thoughts are means by which we attain our objects." My object is to enter into eternal loving relationship with Sri Nama Avatara and, though the journey may be long, I will begin with a first thought of love. This is not "brainwashing" or an artificial mental adjustment. It is a natural process that will take me in any direction that I like. I know my goal and think accordingly. As I think, so shall I feel, and as I feel, so shall I will or desire. When that desire is exceedingly great, then I begin to actually live in the mahamantra.

Just as soon as I become aware of the true situation through direct realization I seem to explode with a burst of loving sentiment for Sri Nama Avatara. This feeling of love, as it could be understood or expressed by material standards, has been referred to in the early stages as *ruci* or *taste* by the great authorities of mahamantra yoga. It is still but a tiny droplet of vapor compared to the ocean of love remaining dormant within the heart. In the beginning the heart sits lifelessly, frozen by the bitter cold of the dense world of matter. Sri Nama Avatara has begun to awaken and melt the true heart and in the very beginning this melting is experienced as the escaping of some particles of vapor. This vapor is very, very sweet. One becomes captivated by the sweetness and in just a short while the former sweetness of the material sensual experience is no longer able to satisfy the true self. Sri Nama Avatara now captures me through the pleasure principle. Only a brief span of material time separates me from total perfection. Sooner or later, depending upon the intensity of my practice and the mercy of Sri Nama Avatara, I will meet my cherished goal.

Point 5.7
Bathe your entire being in the purifying vibration of the mahamantra and directly perceive the resulting purification of your self.

This activity of mentally bathing in the sound vibration of the mahamantra can be practiced before and after the material body is transcended. In the early stages faith acts as the vessel that holds the liquid of the mahamantra. Later, when the spiritual nature of Sri Nama Avatara is disclosed, direct experience is the vessel and the liquid of the mahamantra takes on a very clear, pure, and potent character. In either case, however, purification is taking place. The purification becomes more and more obvious as my hearing and chanting progresses. There is nothing very technical about this point. I simply adopt the mood of bathing in sound vibration.

Point 5.8
Know that due to the powerful presence of Sri Nama Avatara you now mount the threshold of immense life-shattering and life-restructuring spiritual realizations.

This point applies to the situations both before and after one transcends the physical plane of time and space. The difference lies only in the degree of spiritual experience. With each leap on to higher planes, my life is changed to accommodate new elements. Just as one wakes up from the dreams of sleep, so dynamic new perspectives replace the worldviews of my former life.

Before I had experienced the transcendence through the practice of mahamantra yoga, it was difficult to understand the high intensity of the realized states. In the beginning there is the need for faith, but with some perseverance there will be a fruitful reward. The fruit of my perseverance drops into my life as profound spiritual realizations. These lucid spiritual realizations are so essential to effect continuation on the path. One will not be able to continue for very long without some tangible result. A superficial continuation will never satisfy the heart and consequently will never last. I either push onward far upstream to the shores of the internal forest or get carried away downstream to the outer world of the senses.

Results for spiritual practitioners should always be measured by the characteristic of the consciousness that the practices engender. Elevation through the hierarchy of ashrams or management within an institution dedicated to spiritual upliftment should never be the gauge for measuring advancement. Unfortunately we have seen all too often that many who are devoid of deeper spiritual intelligence and dynamic spiritual realizations tread this path of so-called elevation within the ranks of the spiritual order.

The attainment of deep and lasting spiritual realizations should be a primary point of reference for the beginning and intermediate practitioners of mahamantra yoga. Once attained, these realizations should be discussed with other similarly experienced followers. His Divine Grace A. C. Bhaktivedanta Swami Prabhupada has compared such discussions to the deliberations of scientific researchers who, after experimenting, consider their progress and results through confidential verbal exchanges. If one is not allied with such a group of realization-oriented devotees of Sri Nama Avatara, then it becomes necessary to seek out such souls and somehow begin a correspondence with them. Faith builds realization and realization builds faith. Strong spiritual association builds both faith and realization.

Part 2. Expulsive Approach to Intensification

Point 5.9
Expel all traces of material egoism.

This area of discussion has been preliminarily covered in points 2.3 through 2.5. There we dealt with preparatory conceptions and practices that would assist us in our entrance into the transcendence. Here, though it is ultimately not up to us, we are aiming at prolonging our stay in the absolute realm once Sri Nama Avatara has blessed us with what is herein called the profound hearing and chanting of the mahamantra.

There are diverse subtleties involved when discussing states of consciousness. When I employ language in my consideration of ordinary everyday consciousness, I usually find myself at a loss. For millennia great thinkers have grappled with the problem of consciousness and diverse positions are still put forward without any firm conclusions. Some see no end in sight. How then am I to speak about the extraordinary states of consciousness brought about by Sri Nama Avatara that are so drastically different from and so far beyond profane experience? How can the nonrealized soul understand anything at all? Where will that individual's reference point be?

The only way to grasp the significance of these descriptions and techniques is through practice. The realizations await my ardent practice. Despite the shortcomings of language and my inability to use language as a satisfactory method of communication, one thing is clear and sure—intensified practice of mahamantra yoga takes me further and further away from the relative plane of dualistic consciousness.

In the beginning of my realizations of the transcendence it is almost unavoidable that impurities will bubble up from the subconscious levels of the mental plane. After all, I have been associated with the material world for countless eons. The impressions laid to rest upon the mind are numberless. These impurities are all by-products of *ahankara,* the shallow but pernicious sense of ego that causes me to falsely identify with what I am not, to think that mind and body are self. These impurities must be released and expelled in order for me to continue in ecstatic association with the radiance of Sri Nama and later with Sri Nama Avatara Himself.

In a number of places the *Bhagavad-gita* discusses this topic of mental impressions, detachment from desires, and transcendence of the qualities of material nature—*gunas*.

> *apuryamanam acala-pratistham*
> *samudram apah pravisanti yadvat*
> *tadvat kama yam pravisanti sarve*
> *sa santim apnoti na kama-kami*

[Translation:]

A person who is not disturbed by the incessant flow of desires—that enter like rivers into the ocean, which is ever being filled but is always still—can alone achieve peace, and not the one who strives to satisfy such desires.

BHAGAVAD-GITA 2:70

And in the fourteenth chapter one also finds,

> *sri-bhagavan uvaca*
> *prakasam ca pravrttim ca*
> *na dvesti sampravrttani*
> *na nivrttani kanksati*
>
> *udasina-vad asino*
> *gunair yo no vicalyate*
> *guna vartanta ity evam*
> *yo 'vatisthati nengate*
>
> *sama-duhkha-sukhah sva-sthah*
> *soma-lostasma-kancanah*
> *tulya-priyapriyo dhiras*
> *tulya-nindatama-samstutih*

> *manapamanayos tulyas*
> *tulyo mitrari-paksayoh*
> *sarvarambha-parityagi*
> *gunatitah sa ucayate*

[Translation:]

The Supreme Personality of Godhead said: O son of Pandu, he who does not hate illumination, attachment and delusion when they are present or long for them when they disappear; who is unwavering and undisturbed through all these reactions of the material qualities, remaining neutral and transcendental, knowing that the modes alone are active; who is situated in the self and regards alike happiness and distress; who looks upon a lump of earth, a stone and a piece of gold with an equal eye; who is equal toward the desirable and the undesirable; who is steady, situated equally well in praise and blame, honor and dishonor; who treats alike both friend and enemy; and who has renounced all material activities—such a person is said to have transcended the modes of nature.

BHAGAVAD-GITA 14:22–25

If I perceive certain relative conceptions trying to enter the field of my consciousness, I first establish an attitude of neglect toward such conceptions. I do not fight them and do not try to force them out. I gently release through *neglectful witnessing,* much like allowing clouds to float by. I also induce the nondoing attitude of *neglect of neglect.* I remain oblivious to the process of neglect itself. Experience is often the best teacher here as it is with many of the subtleties that have been covered in these pages.

Besides neglect I also pray to Sri Nama Avatara and His many representatives to help me to remain identified as nonmaterial atomic sentience. Any sense of prayer will be very deep and powerful once having crossed the threshold of spiritual realization. One may pray, "Dear Lord, now appearing before me in your divine incarnation as the Holy Names, please free me from the contractions of this sense of material ego." Sri

Nama Avatara will certainly help one, and through His grace one will be given other means in addition to the mental process of neglect and the devotional act of prayer for conquering the lower self.

Point 5.10
Expel all attitudes tending toward exploitation of Sri Nama Avatara such as desires for self-aggrandizement, sexual intercourse, and various other mundane pursuits.

Sri Nama Avatara is the master and I am the servant. Is the service of the servant meant for satisfying the servant's desires or for satisfying the master's desires? Sri Nama Avatara is not like some tool at my disposal meant to bring about the gratification of my material desires. My association with Sri Nama Avatara is meant for His pleasure. When the master is satisfied, then the servant is automatically satisfied, just as the bodily limbs feel nourishment when foodstuffs are channeled toward the stomach.

Here within point 5.10 are some examples of the various impurities that can seep in to my field of consciousness. The two specific ones mentioned—desire for name and fame, and desire for sexual intercourse—form for many individuals the basis of their internal thought programs within the consensus reality. The latter of these two, desire for sexual intercourse, is hardwired into the physical body for the perpetuation of the species. This makes it a powerful obstacle for one who remains identified with the body. The desire for name and fame is a subtle aspect of the mental body and thus a challenge for those who are more identified with the mind. There have been many cases of chanters of the mahamantra who were completely diverted by these two elements of programming. Be very much on guard against these two aspects of the false ego's infestation.

Sri Nama Avatara can bring anything to me. I approach Sri Nama Avatara for only the purest end—Krishna-prema—pure, eternal, limitless love of Godhead. Just as a surgeon would not use his finest scalpel to chisel wood, so I will not misuse the powers of the mahamantra for the acquisition of material ends.

Point 5.11
Expel all thoughts of time, speed of recitation, numbers, and other calculative conceptions.

These calculative conceptions as well as others not mentioned here are contaminants that are to be avoided as far as possible. The mere thought to enjoy the taste of foodstuffs not yet offered to Krishna spoils the offering of an advanced devotee. Similarly, while serving the holy names of Krishna, one must steer clear of all forms of contaminating calculative mentality.

As I enter the transcendence through the grace of the mahamantra, I find that external thoughts no longer plague me. The experience is so powerful. Still, my association with the Supreme Pure is but a new birth, while my association with matter—an old illness. Due to that material intimacy, sometimes I feel that calculative tendencies are pushing in on me. I expel such tendencies and keep them at a distance by deepening my meditation on the ever-sweetening sound vibration that is now engulfing me.

Point 5.12
Expel all chanting methods that create distractions to mahamantra meditation.

In memory I span the years that I have been attempting communion with the transcendental sound vibration, and I recall many types of approach that did not help me. Though my intentions may have been sincere, the results were not perceivably good ones. There was a time that I chanted while standing and facing the wall in the corner of a room. I would sway, move my head from side to side, and chant the mahamantra. There were other times that I would go on walks in natural settings and chant. I have tried chanting while referring simultaneously to certain verses of *sastra*. I have also tried moving my head back and forth while sitting. I have bobbed and bounced and shaken. I have sought so many means to somehow hear the sound of the mahamantra and get through the last round of my numerical vow of rounds. Though I have not gone the extra step to procure the small metal counting devices for keeping count of one's rounds (a measure that seems to result in only the most distracted kind of chanting imaginable), I must admit that I have considered acquiring such a device.

There is one incident that comes to mind when reflecting upon this topic of poor methods of hearing and chanting. This incident occurred in Bombay (present-day Mumbai) sometime in the early 1970s. A number of devotees were chanting on their beads in a room that was serving as a makeshift temple. Many were undergoing the aforementioned rigors of distracted hearing and chanting. Some paced back and forth. Some bobbed. Some swayed in corners. Some shook their heads while others shook their beads. Suddenly without any announcement, the spiritual master appeared on the scene. He sat down and began chanting on his beads. In less than two or three minutes all the former commotion had ceased. Everyone was sitting and chanting "properly." Merely by the presence and example of the pure devotee of Sri Nama Avatara, all the rubbish methods had been put out in one sweep.

Having seen the example of my spiritual master as well as pictures and descriptions of earlier pure devotees of Sri Nama Avatara, I can now say that despite trying so many unusual means, I really knew deep within the correct way to hear and chant. The correct way is the commonsense way. Only mental weakness delivered me to the wrong methods. "How am I to chant and hear so that the mahamantra is the sole content of my consciousness?" By answering this question honestly within my heart, I am delivered to the correct method.

Once I have been granted entrance into the transcendence through the practice of intensified hearing and chanting of the mahamantra, my earlier approaches seem unintelligent and actually in opposition to the principle of intensified hearing and chanting.

Point 5.13
Expel tendencies toward enjoyment of the new and wondrous inner domains of consciousness revealed by Sri Nama Avatara.

The mahamantra takes me to new realms never before visited. The true nature of those realms surpasses the shallow ideas that profane consciousness may produce about them, much like a visit to the ocean surpasses a mere description of the ocean. The mood of enjoyment must not be carried over into those realms. We arrive in those spaces by our attitude of surrender and service. Freedom from the selfish enjoying mood characterizes realized states. I must keep on guard to bar all moods of enjoyment from my consciousness, even though I have habituated myself to adopt such moods over many lifetimes of existence within the material worlds. I have experienced on numerous occasions the deterioration of this great gift of realization by the entrance of an enjoying mood. I will make my goal love of Godhead not the attainment of mystical sensations.

I am reminded of the words of St. John of the Cross in *Dark Night of the Soul:*

> For they think that all the business of prayer consists in experiencing sensible pleasure and devotion and they strive to obtain this by great effort wearying and fatiguing their faculties and their heads and when they have not found this pleasure they become greatly discouraged thinking that they have accomplished nothing. Through these efforts they lose devotion and spirituality, which consists in perseverance, together with patience and humility and mistrust of themselves, that they may please God alone. For this reason when they have once failed to find pleasure in this or some other exercise, they have great disinclination and repugnance to return to it, and at times they abandon it.

I will not seek the bliss of spiritual life like the materialist seeks the gratification of his senses. And when such bliss is bestowed upon me, I shall be careful not to devour it like the hungry animal devours his food.

Point 5.14
Expel all artificially forced mental approaches to Sri Nama Avatara:
1) By expressing deep faith in the mercy and potency of the maha-

***mantra, and 2) By cultivating humility, devotion, service attitude,
patience, reverence, and love.***

"Artificially forced mental approaches" means those approaches to Sri
Nama Avatara that are not founded upon deep faith in Him. I cannot
overemphasize the importance of expressing deep faith in the reality of
Sri Nama Avatara while chanting the mahamantra. This has certainly
been one of the most effective elements in my practice of mahamantra
yoga, and without a doubt the expression of faith and the capacity to
abide in faith would not have been possible had I not cultivated, at least
to some degree, humility, devotion, service attitude, patience, reverence,
and love. These qualities arise in one who attentively follows the path of
bhakti. The necessity of acquiring these qualities through adherence to
the path of bhakti is confirmed by guru, sadhu, and sastra.

It is evident here (just as when studying the ten offenses to Sri
Nama Avatara that are described in the *Padma Purana*) that a twenty-
four-hour program is necessary. My endeavors in mahamantra yoga go
beyond the immediate time that I am directly hearing and chanting.
The actions and thoughts that occur throughout the other times of the
day and night play an important role in my approach to the incarnation
of the Godhead as sound.

I seek to get more and more strength by associating with pure devotees of Sri Nama Avatara—directly if possible (*vapu*) and through their
sound vibration (*vani*). The sound vibration presence and association
of the pure devotees is considered the more important of the two features of sadhu-sanga, and it can be had readily in these times by reading
authorized books of spiritual culture in the association of more advanced
devotees and with other sincere candidates for spiritual advancement. If
there is one single type of activity that will help me, it is the valuable
activity of associating with saintly persons (sadhu-sanga), and all great
spiritual authorities have repeatedly emphasized this truth.

I will now thank you for your time and patience. I have asked much
from you as the reader, and you have tolerated much to come this far

with me. In the final analysis my motives for writing this book may not be knowable. However, I can say with some degree of certainty why I did *not* write this book. I did not write this book merely for the mental stimulation of its readers. This book has been written to serve as a tool for practice—*intensified* practice—*my* intensified practice and perhaps your intensified practice. Hopefully the readers of this book will seriously attempt the intensified practice of mahamantra yoga following these and other authoritative guidelines. Mental stimulation is useless unless it motivates us to action.

Those who have been involved with the process previously without sufficient intensity, or with diminished intensity, may, upon trying to apply the points of this book, discover that unwanted old habits and ingrained patterns of thought about the practice can be difficult to break or change. This group will have to try much harder and with an even more critical view. It may seem like hard work, but when we look back after having tasted the fruit of living mahamantra yoga, we will think that the price paid was a small one indeed.

Let us all help one another and practice mahamantra yoga with ever-increasing intensity and a pronounced attitude of service and devotion. The service attitude is absolutely essential. Sit firmly with straight back. See nothing and feel tiny. Forget plans but expect something wonderful. Focus the mind and, in due course, hear the infinite loving Godhead within the internal forest of your deeper heart.

हरे कृष्ण हरे कृष्ण

6 Realizations

A look into some of the dramatic and
highly positive transformations of
personal consciousness that occur
during intensified mahamantra yoga

*You must realize my friend, that the deeper we go into this,
both written and spoken words of formal language become
less and less adequate as a medium of expression.*

MANUEL CORDOVA RIOS

This chapter describes some of the subjective experiences that one
may encounter at the dawning of genuine association with Sri Nama
Avatara, the living mahamantra. The initial state of these realizations is herein referred to as entrance into the internal forest of the
heart through the profound hearing and chanting of the mahamantra.
When this occurs, material time and space as well as material egoism fade into oblivion. One contacts the infinitesimal nature of the
true self. A strong and pronounced shift of consciousness becomes
the obvious manifestation, as the practitioner helplessly falls headlong
into a swoon of intense wonder.

In reading this chapter I will clearly understand that these points do not express conceptions of ordinary happiness or common well-being. Those ordinary states are limited to the relative plane. Factual realization is understandable only to the realized. There, within that sacred space of realization, I can know with absolute certainty just what is being described within this chapter. Mere words cannot convey the dynamics and the intensity of realized states of consciousness. Neither the author's articulation nor the reader's sensitivity can help now. Only intensified practice and the mercy of the transcendental agents can provide the full revelation that I desire.

Still, these points have been presented, and further I am attempting to relay some sense of understanding by giving a more detailed description of the subjective characteristics related to these points. It should be emphasized that the points of this chapter have been drawn out of immediate and authentic experience and composed at a later time from memory and from a body of notes. The notes were written down directly after the experiences during a period of more than twenty years. Though I am a very ordinary fellow by material standards, I did in fact on numerous occasions directly perceive and live through all that is about to be described. I do not live continuously in those rarefied states of consciousness, but I have full confidence that I will enter within those wondrous domains and far beyond them in due course when I have become sufficiently purified. I have been *there,* and anyone else who is sufficiently committed can go there as well. Great hope shines down upon all of us. The invitation is extended forever. As mentioned by Srila Bhaktisiddhanta Saraswati Thakura in his forward to *Sri Brahma-samhita,* "The Transcendental Autocrat is ever inviting the fallen conditioned souls to associate with Him through devotion or eternal serving mood." The author of *Mahamantra Yoga* is far less qualified than most other persons. The only conclusion to be arrived at by analyzing all these facts can be stated in the following points:

Point 6.1
That state of profound hearing and chanting of the mahamantra arises by the power and mercy of the mahamantra.

The plane of glory has descended into direct experience. I am delivered to the state of autonomy and freedom from the prison of material conceptions. Now I have passed from the profane into the sacred. I have transcended the relative dualities of matter. I taste the limitless and the eternal. True devotional life has now begun.

> *brahma-bhutah prasannatma na socati na kanksati*
> *samah sarvesu bhutesu mad-bhaktim labhate param*

[Translation:]

> One who is thus transcendentally situated at once realizes the Supreme Brahman. He never laments nor desires to have anything; he is equally disposed to every living entity. In that state he attains pure devotional service unto Me.
>
> BHAGAVAD-GITA 18:54

I see that I possess no special qualities for acquiring entrance within these states of transcendence, and to the contrary, having arrived there, I feel quite unworthy. Though this book has seemingly presented some mechanism or technique for gaining access to the transcendental sphere, once one arrives in that wondrous domain, it becomes evident that some kind of excellent and marvelous grace has bestowed a great blessing.

I feel deeply that my understanding of certain details of the interrelationship between matter and spirit (*jnana*) has not been the cause. I also feel that my immediate detachment from sensual experience has not been the cause. I cannot pinpoint a cause. I cannot trace out a starting point for this thing. I am left only with reflections upon the state of my heart and the nature of my desires.

In chapter 14 of *The Nectar of Devotion,* His Divine Grace A. C. Bhaktivedanta Swami states:

Some scholars recommend that knowledge and renunciation are important factors for elevating oneself to devotional service. But actually that is not a fact. Actually, the cultivation of knowledge or renunciation, which are favorable for achieving a footing in Krishna consciousness, may be accepted in the beginning, but ultimately they may also come to be rejected, for devotional service is dependent on nothing other than the sentiment or desire for such service. It requires nothing more than sincerity.

Point 6.2
That state of profound hearing and chanting of the mahamantra is the dawning of the tireless stage of mahamantra meditation and practice.

Now I can understand what could not be understood before. The idea of ceaselessly chanting the mahamantra has become reality. As a flag is whipped and frayed by strong winds, so is my tongue driven by Sri Nama Avatara. As great underground rivers gush their crystalline pure contents, so the mahamantra forces entrance through the passages of my ear holes, carving gorges within.

Oh my will, where have you gone? Perhaps you still exist somehow, but within my life you are utterly disconnected. My tongue, lips, jaw, and mind—all are carried along effortlessly by the surging currents of the great flowing river of Sri Nama Avatara. This experience is the essence of tireless and ceaseless chanting. All effort has run away. The harsh whip of my intelligence has been cast aside. The beatings so relentlessly carried out upon my mind have ceased. My ears, tongue, and mind have been invited to a festival within the internal forest. There within the shining bowers momentum and strength have become the guards, and my guru maharaja the festival's host. Joy, eternity, cognition, and wonder are some of the amazing guests. *Bhava* and *prema* are scheduled to arrive soon. Feeling unwanted, social convention and material conception have run far away, and no one seems to care.

There is but one drink within this shining bower and pure, simple faith serves it. This drink has taken control of everything, and it seems to cause a kind of madness. This unusual beverage so exquisitely mixed is the profound hearing and deep chanting of the mahamantra and its influence is most intoxicating.

By now so many things have become clear. Sri Nama Avatara is the supreme Subject and I am the tiny object. An object does not tire. An object does not feel the rigors of time. I surrender to the Sound, and He flows through my being. Sri Nama Avatara is chanting me! He is active, dominant. I am passive, open, receptive. This is the reality, and here I find the simple purpose of my existence.

Point 6.3
That state of profound hearing and chanting of the mahamantra reveals all desires for self-aggrandizement and conquest of the world as utterly foolish and vain.

Sri Nama Avatara reveals my true size. I am but a microbe, a mote of life, encased within a minuscule flesh body, moving about on a speck of dust, suspended within a vast black abyss. As things extreme acquire significance, so my extreme tininess might account for something, but I ask, what is the value in becoming a king of germs? Oh Sri Nama Avatara, through your grace, I have glimpsed a fragment of Your splendor and have tasted the wonder of real birth—the dawning of relationship with You, *sambhanda*. How could I want anything else but Your association at a time like this? Those who, whether subtly or grossly, seek worldly name and fame, mundane power and glory, reveal plainly to their inner hearts just how distant they are from you.

Point 6.4
That state of profound hearing and chanting of the mahamantra is relished by the chanter in the way cool, sweet water is relished by a half-dead victim of the desert.

Thirst of the soul has far greater import than any degree of bodily thirst. Forgive me, but point 6.4 is only pale analogy. Metaphor and analogy cannot possibly touch the precincts of Sri Nama Avatara.

Now essence is touched by substance. I am united with the stuff of my being, and that stuff is joy. Prior to Your advent, how could I know such joy? Sri Nama Avatara, You are manifest before me like a great merciful rain cloud and You:

> . . . *extinguish the blazing fire of material existence.*
>
> Sri Sri Siksastaka, verse 1,
>
> by Sri Chaitanya Mahaprabhu

Point 6.5

That state of profound hearing and chanting of the mahamantra engulfs and finally drowns the chanter by a powerful surge of nectar.

The nature of this experience pushes me far past the realms of verbal expression. Prose descriptions are grossly inadequate, while even inspired poetry falls short of my intention. What art, what means of expression could come close to capturing this? Experience is the only medium that is possibly acceptable, and now Your radiance overflows the boundaries of my experience.

The living ocean of Sri Nama Avatara has blown its cooling nectarous spray upon me. I have hardly touched the rim of this living ocean, but still I marvel at the character of its mist. My wonder increases, for I know that the great, purified souls swim freely, diving and surfacing in this deep living ocean at every moment.

The mist of the living ocean hisses within my ears and heightens their ability to perceive sound vibrations. The mist is sweet and cooling. This divine mist gradually thickens and engulfs my being. I stand alone and quietly tremble. Are others with me as I drown in the nectarous mist of the living ocean? Oh Sri Nama Avatara, please let me drown in Your existence while in the association of the nonenvious devotees.

Point 6.6

That state of profound hearing and chanting of the mahamantra causes the chanter to feel the inadequacy of his one tongue and two ears.

Can the great rivers in the monsoon season, fed by torrential rains, be asked to enter into a single receptacle? Can the sky be brought down within the ceiling of my study and expected not to exceed those limits? Can the fierce winds of the cyclone be compressed and forced to pass through the tiny door of my mind? Tiny and fleshy tongue, do you think that your surface is sufficient for the limitless Personality of Godhead to make His dance? Little ear holes, how can the infinite pass through you?

Our great and powerful guru, Srila Rupa Goswami, has said in his *Vidagdha-madhava* (1.15):

> I do not know how much nectar the two syllables "Krs-na" have produced. When the holy name of Krishna is chanted, it appears to dance within the mouth. We then desire many, many mouths. When that name enters the holes of the ears, we desire many millions of ears. And when the holy name dances in the courtyard of the heart, it conquers the activities of the mind, and therefore all the senses become inert.

I am just beginning to comprehend the meaning of Srila Rupa Goswami's statement.

Point 6.7
That state of profound hearing and chanting of the mahamantra thoroughly astounds the chanter.

Wonder! Intense wonder floods my being! The majesty and dimensions of Sri Nama Avatara astound me. I swim in a state of marvelous surprise. This surprise strikes me as being the difference between faith and experience. In the past I have believed in Sri Nama Avatara, but now, as I *live* in Sri Nama Avatara, a reckless thrill races through my heart. What else could result when the infinitesimal is brushed by the infinite? Awestruck, I am poised on the brink of utter devastation.

Point 6.8
Then the power and mercy of Sri Nama Avatara is ushered into the chanter's experience by Sri Nama Avatara Himself.

Now I am made aware of the magnitude and the gift. When such awareness dawns, the cause is not discernible. Yet, I feel outside influences. These influences are so personal and loving. My spiritual master smiles down upon me. Oh Sri Nama Avatara, You are so very personal. Please forgive me that I ever believed You to be less. How could the ordinary mind ever grasp this truth?

Point 6.9
Then perceptions of the initial category of transcendence (brahman) are easily revealed through that power and mercy.

I enter eternity and experience liberation from the death plane. I am a speck in the midst of the endless, timeless sound vibration of Sri Nama Avatara. He shows me a facet of His basic condition, the all-time-presence state of His true environment. This realization is considered insignificant by advanced devotees, and I now can understand that attitude, for I seem to have acquired with ease this positioning beyond durative time—a boon that takes other less fortunate seekers without the grace of Sri Nama Avatara many lifetimes to acquire. I no longer care if anyone believes me or not, for the old me has evaporated.

The sages have propagated the most valuable teachings of mahamantra yoga, but how many have been able to deeply believe in their words? I am mere dirt compared to the acaryas of the mahamantra. My experiences up to now are less than a drop in the sea of joy—the ocean of limitless love, Krishna-prema. A debt of unimaginable proportions has been established. A strong urge to repay this debt wells up from my heart. Surely this is an impossible undertaking. How can I repay my spiritual master for taking me this far? Yet I have no doubt that he will take me further. Some could think I have covered a great distance, but I know that this little bit of realization, though in some way significant, is just the beginning. This stage has been described as containing only a small value when compared to what lies ahead. Oh Treasure of treasures, I have just reached Your static state and await invitation into the dynamic dimensions of absolute services. The exaggeration has not been framed that can come close to Your actual glories.

anayase bhave-ksaya, krsnera sevana
eka Krishna-namera phale pai eta dhana

[Translation:]

As a result of chanting the Hare Krishna mahamantra, one makes such great advancement in spiritual life that simultaneously his material existence terminates and he receives love of Godhead. The holy name of Krishna is so powerful that by properly chanting even one name, one very easily achieves these transcendental riches.

SRI CHAITANYA-CARITAMRTA,
ADI-LILA 8.28

Point 6.10
Then one becomes whole by Sri Nama Avatara's influence and realizes the pure spiritual self as well as utter distinction from all categories of material phenomena.

The conglomeration of gross and subtle matter that I have so long considered to be self has been burned up by these realizations. Senses, mind, wants, intellect—all are pushed aside to reveal a unified, individual, eternal consciousness possessed of attributes that do not belong to the relative world of material time and space. All that I have known is now destroyed. Mother, father, happiness, sadness—the tempest of the world with its names and conceptions—all are completely obliterated within my new absolute worldview.

I have now traveled beyond arguments into the pure state of the proven. Material ideas cannot touch me. I am controlled by powers far too great to be moved to any other views. The tiny feather floating in the wake of a colossal ship can do nothing else but follow, at least for a while. Oh great ship of Sri Nama Avatara, please do not pass me by too quickly.

Point 6.11
Then any doubts about the supreme reality of Sri Nama Avatara are destroyed at their roots.

As Absolute Reality touches me, how can I doubt? Within ordinary experience do I doubt the sun shining upon my head or the earth upon which I stand? My perception of these things, though founded in illusion, builds a flawless faith in their existence. Now I am the subject of a wonderful new kind of perception that has substance, immense substance, and this new kind of experiencing pulls a feeling of shame out of my heart. I do not doubt your supreme reality any longer Sri Nama Avatara. Please forgive me that I ever considered You to be something like ordinary sound. You are beyond my descriptive abilities. I do not feel fit to offer suitable prayers of glorification to You, though I strongly feel the need to do so.

Point 6.12
Then Sri Nama Avatara—the realized form of the mahamantra—becomes the living, acting, directing, Godhead within one's life, bringing Life into life.

Sri Nama Avatara, You have made me live. Before, I only sank in what seemed to be a world dominated by dissolution, the chaotic realm of material time and space that glitters with a mere illusion of life. Before, I was but a superficial person. Oh Sri Nama Avatara, You are so very much alive—You live and act in mysterious ways. Why have you blessed me with this experience of Your deeper realities?

The functioning of my ears has superseded the seeing capacity of my eyes. Your transcendental sound presence has eclipsed all visual categories. You enter my life and direct me. You are working and controlling the movements of all your devotees. My guru maharaja speaks to me through You. You enlighten me and are capable of bestowing material boons upon me. Now I do not care for inert matter, I only want involvement with You.

Sri Nama Avatara, You act in very direct and noticeable ways. You are the source of all knowledge and are very, very personal. Within this amazing material world, very few living beings know these things about you. May you kindly bestow these truths of your reality upon many, many more sleeping souls.

Point 6.13

Upon entering the internal forest by the profound hearing and chanting of the mahamantra, one falls flat before Him, knowing that He, Sri Nama Avatara, is the great shelter of all living beings.

I now attempt to glorify You, Sri Nama Avatara. I know that the limitless living entities who are bound up within the matter of this dark world can be freed by You. I surrender to You, Sri Nama Avatara, and as I do, tears flood these flesh eyes. This flesh throat is choked up by Your influence, and this flesh tongue sputters and struggles to shape Your framework of sound vibration.

Sri Nama Avatara, You possess an absolute form that is wonderfully the same as Your supreme existence as divine sound. Though I have not yet seen that form within my heart, I have heard the authoritative descriptions of that form. Your form has the appearance of a gorgeous young boy. This young smiling boy glows with the all-cognizant light of eternity—a light of which I am but a tiny particle. This form of Yours has a dark bluish color of limitless character and quality. This form is endowed with limbs—two arms and two legs. Beautiful feet carry that form, and the relentless gravity known in this material world does not act upon them. Those beautiful feet have been compared to the lotus flower, and they are very soft and delicate. The soles of those lotuslike feet are of a spiritual pinkish color and are constantly being served by your internal pleasure potency, Srimati Radharani.

This luminous atom of your divine aura flies in the ship of desire to the proximity of the underside of those glorious feet and prays to Sri Radha to be given service in Her camp. Please allow this infinitesimal particle to evolve a spiritual form suitable for serving You.

Point 6.14

Thus one gains powerful convictions and bold determinations to give the living mahamantra to others, to free them of the woes of phenomenal existence within matter.

I now experience some of the truth and glory of Sri Nama Avatara.

Through this experience I am free, and even if I drift out of this consciousness, I now know that I will again enter within it in due course. The end of the night is near. The sun of the mahamantra is now rising within my heart. Still I am aware of the presence of countless other living entities that have not received the shelter of Sri Nama Avatara. Some have not had any exposure, while others, having had some degree of exposure, do not wholeheartedly believe in Him. What are the characteristics of belief, and what is it that causes one to believe before experience has given its blessings?

Now within this moment I have become a real sadhu. Now my words hold conviction and are able to penetrate the minds of those who are unaware of this realm. Tomorrow I may again be a fool, like before, but for now, as I float within the streams of joy and glory of Sri Nama Avatara, I know something of what it is to be a sadhu. Material pride and ego do not act now. One is made a holy person not by one's own doing but by having some contact with the Supreme Holy. This experience awakens the *sadhu* who resides within the still peace of the internal forest of the heart. I am that sadhu. All persons are sadhus within the internal forest of their hearts. Sri Nama Avatara can make everyone a holy person.

Whoever will speak with me now at this moment of realization will believe in Sri Nama Avatara and sense the wonders of His existence. Am I infested with attitudes of pride, vanity, and the desire for name and glory? Some might think such things after hearing these words. But know that the credit goes to Sri Nama Avatara and not to me. I am too small to contain even the slightest amount of credit.

Sri Nama Avatara orders me to give His association to everyone I meet. This is Sri Chaitanya Mahaprabhu's order as well as my spiritual master's. I will extend my help to everyone. Despite the favorable or unfavorable circumstances of my material life, I know that I will struggle again and again to give the mahamantra to the suffering living entities within the world of duality. I can never let my associates think for a moment that this mahamantra is ordinary sound, some dead vibration that sputters out from the flesh fibers within the throat. Sri Nama

Avatara lives, directs, enlightens, and loves. Sri Nama Avatara possesses ultimate and infinite personality.

Point 6.15
All problems are rendered insignificant upon entering into the profound hearing and chanting of the mahamantra.

What are my problems but little ripples breaking against my material body and mind? What are my problems but foul smells having relation only to the foul-smelling contraction known as ego? At this moment those little things are gone and mean nothing. Before coming this far on the path, how could I have ever known freedom from all problems?

Does the ant care as it drowns in the vat of sugar syrup? For an eternal living entity drowning in this sweet, sweet sound of the mahamantra, what is the problem? My body stands in this particular spot within the congregation. The mahamantra surges into the ear holes and tears at the circumferences. There are no problems.

Point 6.16
The mercy and ecstatic revelation of Sri Nama Avatara may be known sometimes even to neophyte chanters.

I am the neophyte chanter by any kind of calculation. My direct experience at this time is proof of point 6.16. It will be up to other neophytes to acquire this proof for themselves. Our great acarya, Srila Rupa Goswami, has confirmed this point in his *Bhakti-rasamrta-sindhu,* text 238.

> *duruhadbhuta-virye'smin sraddha durestu panchake*
> *yatra svalpo'pi sambandha sandhiyan bhava-janmane*

[Translation:]

> Five kinds of devotional activities—namely residing in Mathura, worshipping the Deity of the Lord, reciting Srimad-Bhagavatam, serving a devotee, and chanting the Hare Krishna mahamantra— are so potent that a small attachment for any one of these five items can arouse devotional ecstasy even in a neophyte.

I need only to be sincere, have faith in the reality of the mahamantra, depend upon the mercy of the spiritual masters, cultivate a sincere service attitude, and expect the revelation of Sri Nama Avatara at every moment.

Point 6.17

Upon reaching the internal forest by the path of profound hearing and chanting of the mahamantra, ecstatic transformations of the physical body occur spontaneously.

Like pulses of electrical energy, the hairs of my entire body stand on end and surge back and forth over its surface from head to toe. Tears flood my eyes even though I try to repress them. My throat and voice choke up, and I am unable to enunciate the thirty-two syllables of the mahamantra. Externally, the sound is often unclear, although I strain to correctly pronounce the mahamantra with my tongue and lips.

Again and again my entire body shivers in mysterious waves of joy. Oh, most dear Sri Nama Avatara, what are You going to do with this material body? Perhaps it will tear or explode. Maybe it will melt and run off through the cracks in the floor, or perhaps it might stiffen and remain immobile. I feel the other possibility that my limbs could at any second violently erupt into a furious volley of muscular contractions resulting in a most unusual display of dancing.

My dear Lord, Sri Nama Avatara, I do not take you cheaply. You are the Agent causing forceful bursts of spiritual emotion to rise up from within the depths of my being. I am not to blame. The surge is too powerful, and I cannot check this situation. Do with this body what You will. Thy will be done!

Point 6.18

Upon reaching the internal forest by the path of profound hearing and chanting of the mahamantra, one is unable to return to his birthplace, home, family, or society.

Society, friendship, home, and love—what are these things but illusory mental constructs dependent upon material circumstances for their particular shape and temporary existence? Sri Nama Avatara, You have shattered the plane of mental conceptions and thus You have killed my father and mother, You have destroyed my nation, community, gender, and race. Emotions based upon things and persons related to this physical body have evaporated as would a thin film of moisture in the hot summer sun.

Queer feelings of nostalgia hover about me. Surely these feelings are the remnants of the subtle attachments to my past material relations. In a flash the last traces of these feelings are whisked away by Sri Nama Avatara. Perhaps these mental relations will again become prominent within my life, but for now I am cut off from the world. The peace of pure goodness fills my life. A quiet descends. I exist within the pulse of divine sound. At this present moment my renunciation is complete. I have entered the internal forest. Glory, eternal glory to Sri Nama Avatara!

Point 6.19
Upon reaching the internal forest by the profound hearing and chanting of the mahamantra, all one's relative world conceptions meet with utter destruction.

Dear Sri Nama Avatara, my existence has been reduced to its most basic components, and I know that You are the Agent of this reduction. I am stripped and stand naked before You. You have shown me that life's purpose, whether imagined or factual, becomes life's hub. How wonderful and refreshing to now see before me my simple and true purpose. Within eternity I am to associate with, serve, love, and adore You, Sri Nama Avatara. My dear material mind, I know how odd this statement must sound to you. Though you are not able, please, just try to understand that material conceptions generated by you will never be able to approach Sri Nama Avatara nor give comprehension of the true satisfaction that results from association with Him.

My beneficent Lord, You reduce the material ego in every way. In Your sound vibration incarnation You obliterate all material conceptions, the very building blocks of false ego. Material conceptions are darkness and You are light. Where there is light there can be no darkness. Where

You are present there can be no material conception. May Your rays of glory shine forever in the hallways of my life.

Point 6.20
The brilliant effulgence of Sri Nama Avatara is bursting through my small window! What is a window of light in comparison to the sun?

Dear Sri Nama Avatara, I know that I have not met You in Your entirety. However You have very graciously allowed a portion of Your dazzling and penetrating rays to bless my life. Thus I have been able to see myself for the first time. With the boon of this vision I can understand that greater and greater quantities of Your magnificent splendor will flood my days, and before long I will converse with You in one of the five primary *rasas*. I am sure of this.

I am so tiny, my dear Lord. You are so extensive and boundless. My insignificance makes me a poor receptacle for Your magnificence. Why do You bother to illuminate this modest cup? This little crystal of consciousness that projects out from the void, this speck that I am, thanks You sincerely.

Point 6.21
Oh fortunate living beings, hearers of the eternal glories of Sri Nama Avatara, know for certain that those glories are limitless! Indeed, how much can atomic sentience say about Him? Here this tiny soul Sridhara dasa has minutely reflected the vast, illuminating, and extremely beautiful radiance of Sri Nama Avatara.

My life's experiences are like a mirror, and that mirror is coated with the stuff of words, memories, hopes, and dreams. I am but a small, irregular mirror reflecting a scant portion of the wonders of Sri Nama Avatara. That is all I can do for now. Surely as mirrors of lesser quality produce distorted images due to various irregularities, so the irregularities of material motives must distort my mirrorlike character.

Please bless me, dear reader, and do not condemn me. I have only tried to say something about the most wonderful Sri Nama Avatara. Now I request one thing from you. Please believe with deeper and deeper faith that Sri Nama Avatara will touch your life. He will enter it and conquer the whole of it and, mysteriously, you will be left with nothing and yet given everything. He will plunder your world and strip you bare. What can I do to convince you of the truths of the mahamantra? I beg you to please cut down all limited material conceptions about Sri Nama Avatara, open your heart to Him, and thus meet Him within your heart in no time.

I have worked to discover the reasons why I felt impelled to write this book. Thus far I cannot give any single or conclusive reason. It was, I feel, written more for me than for anyone else. But then my motives for doing this thing must be mixed; for how can I say that I have no material motives at this time? The most I can say is that the main force driving this expression has been the insistent urging of Sri Nama Avatara Himself—not in any kind of overt verbal commandments but rather in subtle proddings that became obvious over time. I expect an auspicious outcome.

Time is vast and human affairs both complex and insignificant. Books and their words go on and on, by the millions. Their authors, by and by, melt away within the dusty corridors of human memory. Now I place this work on the mountain of books churned out by all of those strange bony bodies we call humanity. Find, if you can, a spiritual practice that is more sublime than mahamantra yoga. From this perspective I believe your search will be fruitless. Whoever its author and however flawed its presentation, this book and its subject matter are most worthy and needed. May others more fit take up the task of expounding upon the glories of Sri Nama Avatara and clarifying and refining the means of contacting Him.

So let us gather ourselves now. Without any further hesitation let us move deeply into the region of our hearts and discover there the wondrous internal forest of the living mahamantra. May our journeys on the ever-deepening path of intensified and purified mahamantra yoga be enchanted ones and may each be crowned gloriously with all success.

हरे कृष्ण हरे कृष्ण

7 A Brief Sojourn within the Internal Forest

A poetic summary

It is the land of love, sweetness, charm, and beauty—all are synonymous. It is heart-capturing. Our real existence is neither in our knowledge nor our power, but in our heart. Really, our proper identification is with our heart. So, in which direction our heart is moving, that is the all-important factor in our life. It is a heart-transaction.

SRILA B. R. SRIDHARA MAHARAJA

Closing fast the eyes
Allowing not the false self's gaze
My inner eyes alert
Therein resort to dreamscape's haze
There! Primal consciousness, steady, clear!
Walk gently, the bright region of the heart so near

The true and open heart dear friends
Herein lies that soil sublime
The sweet sleeping soil of the internal forest!

Oh mind, drift calmly to the aural channels
Therein solidly fix, utterly transpose
Cross over the false lake of sensation
That perceptual pool of illusion
Sense the self, small as the floating germ
See Chaitanya dance and beckon to all—
Oh, Supreme Godhead of sheer delight!
In rare respect at His feet we fall!
I beg it please—tear away the veils!
Rain down the truths of the Holy Names!

Oh pilgrim of the internal forest
Follower of the subtle stream and wooded trail
Journey humbly, far into the depths
Farther than the common-day conceives
Thrust the mind into that certain contemplation
While ever patient to the breaks of concentration
Returning again to joy's rough path
Sense of being ever shrinking
Finding myself beneath the blades of straw
Smaller! . . . I go smaller without ending
Fast retreating from the six-foot size
"Behold! . . . I am but a minute speck of life!"
Then, without warning—the world descending
My self enveloped by an ocean vast
Ripped out and sucked down into sweet infinity
Sweet, deep infinity!

All that I have heard now shines real!
A star-filled heaven of gems
Clusters upon clusters explode within my heart
Never . . . never let me go!
Let the chant proceed without urging
Bathing in that fathomless treasure
Thus harmonized, with mind unaltered
Humbled by the brilliant truth
Without a care for time or measure
Advance the spirit with certainty!

Oh, the jolting plight of these babes benign
Tiny souls with tortured minds
Still so new to this art sublime
Alas . . . they revert with chanting's end
To human height and cloudy sky
On over into the dim light of plain day
Descending yet within night's cold abyss
Into the pale pulse of blood and bone.

But hear small children!
Little worshippers of the holy sound
Within our hearts,
Forever keep that marvelous key
Know it for certain,
Our internal forests will be found
Unlocked by grace—sweet, deep eternity
Knowledge, Love, and absolute Bliss
Sri Chaitanya's order clear
The simple path to all of this
"More humble than the straw
More tolerant than the tree
Devoid of false prestige

Respecting all others"
Aware of our true insignificance
Then we will truly see
Then we are made right!

Now run the course of the holy chant
Have our steps upon the sylvan trail sublime
Take us there without urging, into light
Into the cool peace of our innermost heart
Meeting, embracing, utterly consumed
And loving the sacred name incessantly!

Oh sweet, deep soil of the internal forest, hold me firm
My roots spread far in thee
Oh Sound Sublime, my dearest loving Friend
Hold me firm
My sweet, deep Infinity.

Hare Krishna Hare Krishna Krishna Krishna Hare
   Hare
Hare Rama Hare Rama Rama Rama Hare Hare

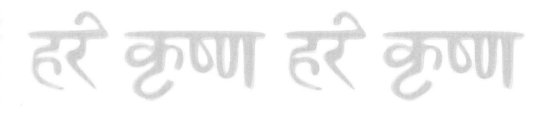

Epilogue

Nature is incomprehensible at first
Be not discouraged, keep on,
There are divine things well envelop'd,
I swear to you there are divine beings
More beautiful than words can tell.

WALT WHITMAN

I completed the manuscript of *Mahamantra Yoga* more than twenty years ago. Looking back, that completion seems to be symbolic of far more than just an end to an exercise in written expression. A significant phase of my life had also come to a close. In a way that I could not have imagined a decade earlier, I found myself striking out on my own and moving away from the shelter of what had become a global institution. Though this move seemed to be a necessity, as the father of a young family I felt greatly challenged by these circumstances.

For those of us who had been fully committed to the demanding lifestyle of mahamantra yoga, the 1977 death of the spiritual master of the worldwide expression of this yoga tradition, Srila A. C. Bhaktivedanta Swami Prabhupada, was experienced as cataclysmic. Unfortunately, it didn't take long for fractures to begin developing in the organization he founded, and for many of his sincere students the application of the pure teachings that he so tirelessly worked to establish seemed to be disintegrating right before their eyes. With each passing year many of his disciples left the familiarity of the institutional life and endeavored to find their way by living in what they considered to be "the outside world."

So in 1990, shortly after the completion of this book, I moved my family from Hawaii to Australia, and to earn a living I sought training in Ericksonian psychotherapy and clinical hypnosis. As a natural outcome of this field of study and after working with many hundreds of clients, I found myself beginning to extend my studies to include research into systems theory, the Gaia hypothesis, the philosophy of mind, and numerous psychological and metaphysical perspectives. In what Castaneda's Yaqui sorcerer don Juan Matus might have described as "a path with heart," I was drawn intensely and systematically for two decades through diverse arenas of human investigation and experience. These included the newly developing field of ecopsychology as expressed by Michael J. Cohen, Ralph Metzner, Paul Shepard, Arne Naess, and Theodore Roszk; shamanic and mythological perspectives as expressed by Joseph Campbell, Robert Lawlor, Douglas Gillette, Jeremy Narby, Carlos Castaneda, and Mircea Eliade; Jungian psychology and the neo-Jungian archetypal psychology of James Hillman, Robert Sardello, and Thomas Moore; the newly emerging field of neurocardiology as broadcast by Doc Childre's HeartMath Institute, Paul Pearsall, Puran Bair, and Joseph Chilton Pearce; the nondual perspectives of Zen, Advaita, Chan Buddhism's Huang Po, and Taoism's Lao Tzu and Chuang Tsu; and modern teachers in some of these areas such as Jean Klein, Franklin Merrell-Wolff, Nisargadatta, Eckhart Tolle, and David Hawkins.

I have been inspired and enriched by the visionary works of numerous writers, teachers, and innovators including Pierre Teilhard de Chardin, Richard Tarnas, Thomas Merton, Herman Melville, Meister Eckhart, John O'Donohue, Robert Temple, Henry David Thoreau, Jach Pursel and Lazaris, Eva Pierrakos, Robert Johnson, Thomas Berry, John Bradshaw, Robert Monroe, Ronald Havens, Gay and Kathlyn

Hendricks, Jean Giono, Guy Murchie, Duane Elgin, Ken Wilber, Ernest Rossi, David Cheek, Brian Swimme, Olaf Stapledon, Jon Kabat-Zinn, Connirae Andreas, David Kennedy, Christian de Quincy, Ron Kurtz, Robert Anton Wilson, Stephen Harrod Buhner, Julian Jaynes, Darryl Anka-Bashar, Paul Levy, John C. Lilly, Milton H. Erickson, Elisabet Sahtouris, Peter Kingsley, and Terence McKenna.

The astounding poetry of Walt Whitman, R. M. Rilke, William Wordsworth, Wendel Berry, Rumi, Pablo Neruda, and haiku giants Basho, Buson, and Issa continues to provide soul nourishment, as do perspectives on natural farming of Masanobu Fukuoka and the masterful accounts of the insect realms given by Maurice Maeterlinck, Simon Buxton, Karl von Frisch, Bert Holldobler, Edward O. Wilson, Jurgen Tautz, and J. E. Lauck. These and other sources not mentioned have not only exposed me to an array of fascinating perspectives, structures of belief, and moving insights but have on occasion exerted a powerful grounding influence upon my continuing development within the human experience.

Though I have mentioned some of the literature of the tradition of mahamantra yoga in the bibliography, I am hoping that this partial list of my past two decades of investigations could for the present-day Western reader serve as a point of reference by which to wade out into the potentially deep waters of mahamantra yoga. From my current perspective, I often catch myself thinking that the teachings of this tradition would be best kept secret, because the extremely esoteric realities of its conceptions are all too easily made into something like the limited stories of the waking dream of this material realm. In what seems like the greatest paradox of all, it is extremely easy to place all of these transcendental teachings into the mundane ego's contexts of duality while barely batting an eye. Indeed most academics do this all the time. Nevertheless, the *acaryas* of mahamantra yoga have consistently wanted this profound work to be disseminated throughout the world, and their sincere followers will endeavor to do this according to the current considerations of time, place, and circumstance. And it is true; superficial investigations are likely to lead one astray. But make no mistake about it.

This tradition of mahamantra yoga is founded upon, grounded within, and saturated by a mentally impenetrable transcendent infinity. Radha and Krishna are calling all of us from that realm—continuously.

The belief structures of this tradition are vast and inclusive of just about all areas of human concern. However in nearly every instance those structures are subordinate to the transcendent experiences of the *bhakta*—the devotee on the path of mahamantra yoga. As with any scientific experiment, if the reader is willing to test the waters by maintaining a glimmer of openness to those conceptual structures and then to try out the practices, there will be an onset not only of the powerful revelations spoken of in this volume but also of far greater revelations that are described in detail throughout the scores of scientific works that have been written in the past five hundred years by the followers of Sri Chaitanya Mahaprabhu.

So what is it that runs this process? What is its fuel? The fuel, the energy source of this spiritual process is causeless mercy itself. The capacity to even believe in the potentials of this process is founded upon causeless mercy. There is really nothing one can *do* to gain access to it. If one is sincerely interested in, or even only slightly curious about, the practices of mahamantra yoga, that causeless mercy will surely enter the life of that individual through the grace of a pure devotee within the lineage. That flow of grace can bring about powerful ontological shifts of perspective that manifest intensely and dramatically, far more dramatically than the familiar scene when Dorothy emerges from her uprooted farmhouse and steps out into the strange and colorful land of Oz.

Advice for total newcomers would be to spend time contemplating from the region of the physical heart both the astounding context of their material life in this vast universe and the dreadful nature of infinity. These two heart-based contemplative exercises as discussed in greater detail in appendix 1 provide an enhanced context for an initial exposure to this tradition's conceptual framework regarding the personality of Godhead, the Godhead's transcendental names, and the supreme realm, Goloka. But then, no matter how we try to frame them, these personal manifestations are so radically beyond our mind's capacity for understanding and so utterly transcendental that even though descriptions may be attempted, the linguistically bound mind remains forever separated from even the slightest glimpse of these divine wonders. Carefully consider, and remember . . . remember . . . if one is thinking about Radha and Krishna and Their divine pastimes in Goloka with the common everyday mind . . . *that* simply is not *It.*

The readers of this book are invited to correspond with me via e-mail. I will work to reply to all who write to me.

richardwhitehurst33@gmail.com

Hare Krishna

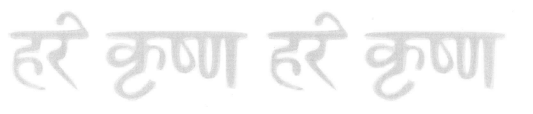

APPENDIX 1

$\mathcal{B}$uilding a Context for Mahamantra Yoga

There are only two ways to live your life. One is as though nothing is a miracle. The other is as though everything is.

ALBERT EINSTEIN

Humanity is adrift upon a marvelous sea of mystery. Though we press onward in the little rowboats of science and technology, this sea continues to expand in every direction far off before us into dim and fading horizons. These horizons, like the proverbial will-o'-the-wisp, recede from us insistently, in step with the evolution of our instruments. Though it seems like we are in the process of acquiring knowledge, we continue to discover that overall we are still merely drifting about in our stories— engulfed by this stupendous and seemingly impenetrable enigma of existence. The surrounding circumstances of immensity and intricacy force us to consider both the limitations of our sensory systems and the inadequacy of language to meet the descriptive demands of this astounding place. We are sorely challenged as we look upon our circumstance with greater and greater refinement. And yet courageously, as individuals and collectively as a species, we press onward, undaunted as we seek our primordial source.

The scales of magnitude stretch from the minute precision of the biochemical realms out into the ineffable vastness of space. The greatest minds of our time are stunned, as the universe looms large in all its magnificent detail. It is this mind-numbing circumstance of the context of our environment that demands an intense engagement of our thoughts, our feelings, and especially our imaginations. The observations of science are utterly astounding, but it would be wrong to assume that we must necessarily be able to comprehend those observations. In his book *The Human Phenomena* the twentieth-century scientist and visionary Pierre Teilhard de Chardin elaborates upon his own reactions to the novelty of these expanding perspectives. There, in a broad way, he categorizes into three basic types of nauseating experiences or "maladies" the effects of actually *seeing* into the variegated enormity of physical reality.

First to be considered here is the malady of the enormity of numbers of things. However, before we can be sickened in dreadful awe by the countless things spread out all around us, we need to recognize and acknowledge how we have been deceived by the very ideas we have about numbers themselves. It is for the most part a self-deception.

The Problem of Numbers

Often without adequate consideration, we learn to talk about large numbers with, at best, a meager understanding of just what they mean and with little or no understanding of their relation to our immediate life circumstances. It is so easy to say "one billion," but a great deal more is required to actually bring that number into a workable conception that has tangible, immediate meaning. As a species moving toward a more comprehensive stage of self-awareness and unification, we need to *see* these magnitudes in our hearts and *feel* them in our guts. Nowadays huge numbers are bandied about by nearly every element of society and, except for extremely rare instances, large numbers roll off our backs devoid of any true comprehension. For the most part we haven't gotten even slightly damp.

In order to appreciate this book's topic, mahamantra yoga, and to approach it in a way that will be more fruitful, it will help to first get saturated within these scales of magnitude. Reasons for this should become clear as we progress. For now if we can embrace our cosmic context we may begin to understand what Teilhard de Chardin is doing when he brings together the concepts of immensity and sickness.

As we move through this appendix, I will ask the reader to slow down at times and work toward the various expansions in thought, feeling, and imagination that are being offered. With patience and a little practice, one will often find oneself in a radically expanded context without having moved an inch. Large numbers require a moment of reflection to actually feel them and to know what they mean. Let us wander slowly through these conceptual realms and spend more time in breaking down really large numbers into more manageable and meaningful pieces.

The Enormity of Numbers of Things

Our lives are nested within so many *things,* and with the discoveries of the past fifty years our awareness of the numbers of things has grown considerably. For example, biologists have catalogued some 1.4 million species. Though many people might think that biologists have for the most part discovered nearly all the species there are, the biologists themselves now know from more recent observations that they have just scratched the surface and have varying estimates of the total number of species on earth that range from 10 to 100 million.*

Advancements in astronomical instrumentation now enable us to

---

*Edward O. Wilson, *The Diversity of Life* (Cambridge, Mass.: Belknap Press of Harvard University Press, 1992).

peer out from far above the earth's atmosphere into the near perfect transparency of space where light that has been traveling for more than thirteen billion years falls within the grasp of ultra-sensitive receivers capable of translating minute streams of photons and other frequencies into the visual images of early galaxies. Based on current observations it has been calculated that in the known universe there are more stars (huge and inconceivably powerful thermonuclear balls of gas) than there are grains of sand on all the beaches of Earth!

Spend a moment now and try to remember the last time you were among grains of sand, and then put these two ideas together. How are we to proceed as we further consider that many of these stars have planets orbiting about them? How are we to get *that* into the marvelous but limited vessels of our minds? Are we not utterly stifled—amazed—by the severity of our circumstance?

The Enormity of Space

This brings us to the second malady—the insidious revelation of the enormity of space. This realm we are in is so inconceivably gigantic that descriptions of its dimensions need to be given in terms of the distance light travels in one year. When we consider extended flights across the Pacific that drag on for hours and the fact that light can travel around the earth nearly eight times in one second, we just might begin to feel ourselves fading. The ninety-three million miles from the earth to the sun are eight minutes by light speed. Think now—and imagine. See this in your mind's eye. One second—eight times around the earth. Eight minutes equals 480 seconds, which equals 3,840 times around the earth. How long does it take to walk one mile? How long would it take to fly the distance from the earth to the sun in a 747 (3,840 times around the earth) . . . or to fly even one light-year at those paltry subsonic speeds?

Maybe "not getting it" is nature's way of protecting the brain—a type of conceptual ceiling that saves us from being overwhelmed by burnout. The brain is structured for perceiving and conceiving at the human scale. I think most readers will agree that as gloriously complex as it is, the brain in its current state will never be able to grasp this cosmic category of enormity. Conceptually most of us can't even grasp in a meaningful way the distance to the moon or the dimensions of the solar system. Even if a "theory of everything" were to eventuate and the nature of physical reality were reduced to a series of mathematical formulations, that will not be *This*. Perhaps Thomas Merton's perspective on the incomprehensible nature of our condition is a wise orientation after all, wherein he says, "Life is not a problem to be solved but rather a mystery to be lived."

The nearest star to our sun is some 4.3 light-years distant. If the sun were the size of a pea, this nearest star would be approximately one hundred miles away. In 4.3 years there are more than 135 million seconds—eight times around the earth in one second—over one hundred million seconds—sun the size of a pea—one hundred miles away. You might take a couple of minutes and notice how it feels to play around with this analogy picturing these elements within your mind as you maintain an understanding that at this scale the entire earth would be microscopic.

Our home galaxy, the Milky Way, is one hundred thousand light-years across. If the sun were shrunk down to the size of the period at the end of this sentence, then by comparison the diameter of the galaxy would be larger than the actual diameter of the earth.* Think of the size of the period at the end of this sentence held up to the size of the world that surrounds you. And . . . humanity is now able to see some thirteen *billion* light-years in every direction with a currently estimated total of between fifty and one hundred billion galaxies. These observations, when deeply considered and not merely brushed over, do in fact bring that peculiar and queasy feeling akin to what is commonly felt when one's life is threatened. If you don't feel that ontological nausea, then consider—if you dare—spending more time in contemplation of these terrible magnitudes. Focus, and go deeper. Be taken.

I remember being in a hurricane in the Florida Keys back in the late

*Ken Croswell, *Magnificent Universe* (New York: Simon and Schuster, 1999).

1980s. Though the gusts were barely more than ninety miles an hour, making it a small storm by hurricane standards, the pressure of those blasts was staggering—literally. I was only just able to maintain my grip on an iron railing along a seawall bordering the Florida Straits. Looking out across those waters as I felt this power that threatened to tear me away, I meditated upon the fact that hurricanes were mere spin-offs of solar radiation and that they had their true origins in the atomic processes of the sun's core. And yet only two-billionths of the total solar output falls upon this planet. When seen from but a few hundred miles above the earth these immensely powerful storms meander across the surface like delicate disks of very slowly rotating cotton. During the twenty minutes I was blasted by those winds I tasted the bitter sweetness of my own insignificance.

The Enormity of Time

The third malady—that of the enormity of durative linear time—is enough to squash even the most ambitious of intellects. We live our lives a few seconds at a time. For most people the occurrence of their life quickly registers in memory as minutes, and then as hours, days, weeks, months, years, and so forth. The moon has gone around the earth well over forty billion times, roughly once every four weeks. Let us meditate upon this. Can we imagine the twenty-four thousand orbits of the moon around the earth since the time of the Roman Empire and the death of Jesus? And do the two thousand years of recent history mean very much to us when we think of the billions of years of the elapsed time of life on earth?

Try performing some mental time travel when you next see the moon hanging in the night sky and know it was there, looking just as it does now, above the first vertebrate that crawled out of the primordial seas of the unconscious. Beneath the cool presence of the orbiting moon, mountain ranges have pressed upward only to be broken down by wind, rain, heat, cold, glaciers, and earthquakes. Continents have drifted apart and crashed into one another. Let us be humbled and reduced as we contemplate these occurrences from the tiny moments of our individual life stories. Boredom becomes impossible in the face of well-imagined geological time. Avoid the temptations and fixations of existential anxiety and instead . . . resort to awe. Our circumstances are truly awe-full.

Entering into the Process

In this rich compost of grandeur we are now perhaps ready to consider the most awe-full of all as we discover ourselves loitering about the outskirts of infinity—an important principle that lies at the very heart of the practice that has just been described—mahamantra yoga. Having warmed up with the three maladies, let us return to our human scales of time and space and from that familiar place peer back into those faint and fading horizons as I attempt to briefly recount my introduction to this ancient tradition.

The time: late November 1970. The space: the north-central Florida peninsula at the University of Florida where I was enrolled as a student. This was the setting of my first exposure to mahamantra yoga, something that turned out to be both powerful and pivotal. In psychological terms what happened to me could be described as a "comprehensive dissociative breakdown of the ego structures." The subjective characteristics of this event however went far beyond any of the verbiage of twentieth-century psychology. My contact with the mahamantra (the great mind-liberating sound vibration) resulted in an astounding insight into the true nature of my identity. Up to that point in my life "I" had been identifying as the mind and the physical body. Through the recitation of the mahamantra I could see with crystal clarity that I was not the mind, nor the physical body, nor the thoughts or feelings associated with these things. Within a mere thirty minutes of practicing the vibration of the mahamantra, I realized my *self* as pure nonconceptual awareness existing outside of linear time and three dimensional space—completely distinct from all categories of material conception. This was an unassailable insight beyond any need for explanations or proofs, and it became a compelling motivation to enter more deeply into the process.

As I involved myself further with the mahamantra what became evident was that *I* had not actually contacted the mahamantra. He, She, or whatever It was had, more accurately, contacted me. Like a vast and benevolent alien presence, the mahamantra seemed to possess a degree of power and personhood that made no sense at all to my conventional ways of thinking. This exotic sound was immensity itself, and yet it was warm, loving, and intimate.

In the weeks and months that followed I would discover the spiritual context from which this ancient yoga process had emerged. An unbroken line of realized masters originating off-planet and in the far distant past had communicated this science through the current of a living oral tradition that has continued to exist into our present time. Today, after nearly forty years of research and practice, mahamantra yoga and its spiritual tradition remain the most astounding and radical system of belief I have ever encountered, possessing a consistent and unifying philosophical framework that embraces all of the really significant mysteries enveloping the human condition.

Sri Chaitanya Mahaprabhu was the spiritual figure who brought this yoga system out from its esoteric obscurity into a bold prominence over five hundred years ago in West Bengal, India. He arranged for the science of this process to be made explicit by instructing his principle disciples to write books about its many facets. The final result of such practice, he said, is not merely a nonconceptual absolute emptiness (or fullness) nor a vague nonparticipatory heavenly residence, but rather it consisted of entrance into a limitless variegated environment of unending, loving reciprocations—exchanges of intense unadulterated love between inconceivable transcendental *persons*.

More than twenty-four hundred years ago the Greek philosopher Aristotle in his work *Physics* said, "It is incumbent on the person who specializes in physics to discuss the infinite, and to enquire whether there is such a thing or not, and if there is, what it is." In Jewish mysticism there is the concept of the *Ein Sof,* the Infinity of the Godhead. There it is said that Infinity is not to be taken casually. It's a dangerous and destructive thing for those who are not sufficiently purified or adequately prepared. The great teachers in that tradition advise that persons take extreme caution if they are attempting to enter the "garden" of infinity.* Yet Sri Chaitanya went even further in his teachings and stated that the Godhead is manifest in its fullest perfection and expression as an *embodiment* of infinite attributes—a transcendental Person with a form composed of infinite existence, infinite knowledge, and infinite bliss, where the aspects of sweetness, charm, beauty, and pleasure eclipse all other considerations of presence, grandeur, and power. He went on to state that this infinite embodiment was inconceivably one *with* everything and yet at the same time distinct *from* everything. And the Infinite, because it possesses infinite potencies, can make itself known even to the infinitesimal. What an astounding conception!

Each of the more than 6.5 billion human beings on this planet has some sense of their existence. They each have some degree of knowledge and some feelings of joy or bliss, however minute. We each possess the same qualities as that absolute Godhead, but only to an infinitesimal degree. What Sri Chaitanya Mahaprabhu revealed through the practice of mahamantra yoga is no less than a means of gaining access to the very realm where that ultimate embodiment of infinite existence, knowledge, and bliss resides and relates. That transcendent sphere of consciousness existing far beyond the enormity of this universe, he declared, is our true home. As atomic specks of consciousness, we belong *there.*

Walt Disney with the limited capacities of his human mind created something wonderful and endearing to millions—magic kingdoms and an array of fun imaginary characters. What could an infinite intellect with limitless creative capacity manifest for the deepest and most extensive expressions of loving exchange? That is the question. And if that infinite One has an inconceivable form, what shape might that be? And

---

*Amir D. Aczel, *The Mystery of the Aleph: Mathematics, the Kabbalah, and the Search for Infinity* (New York: Four Walls Eight Windows, 2000).

. . . does this personality of the infinite Godhead have names? This has all been directly realized by the perfected mahamantra yogis, and it has been described in great detail in their voluminous and rarefied writings.

This personal Godhead is not the result of an anthropomorphic projection by human beings. Rather, human beings are the result of *theopomorphic* projections of the personality of Godhead. In the dream of physical duality and the illusion of tangibility, we imagine that we exist as outrageously complex biochemical forms within a material realm—one head, two eyes, two ears, one mouth, two arms, two hands, two legs, and two feet. The personality of Godhead that Sri Chaitanya Mahaprabhu described is not a psychological or metaphysical "complex" but rather the Godhead exists as the primordial archetypal template— one head, two eyes, two ears, one mouth, two arms, two hands, two legs, and two feet—and resides far beyond the plane of nonconceptual oneness. This fact brings clarity to statements from other ancient traditions wherein it has been said that humans are created "in the image of God"—not metaphorically but literally. This realm where we presently live is a reflection of that realm. Though our physical universe is immense, it is effortlessly made manifest from moment to moment by the infinite creative and sustaining capacities of that divine agency.

Sri Chaitanya Mahaprabhu declared that mahamantra yoga can bring all sincere souls to the threshold of that timeless infinite Reality existing beyond all the dreamlike manifestations of this astounding physical world. In numerous places the Vedic literature of India says that if in this present and difficult age known as the Kali Yuga one wants self-realization and God consciousness then mahamantra yoga is the recommended thing to do. Mahamantra yoga reveals this most confidential knowledge to that individual who is earnestly absorbed in an attitude of service and dedication—*bhakti*—and it delivers that individual in due course to the intensely vital flow of an unending current of infinite love—the nectarous elixir for which the human heart ceaselessly yearns.

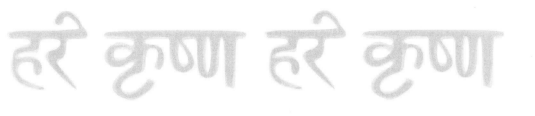

APPENDIX 2

Aphorisms of Mahamantra Yoga

1.1 Eliminate all unnecessary sensory input or stimuli.

1.2 Establish an environment and time for practicing mahamantra yoga.

1.3 Free the environment from external distractions.

1.4 Wear clothing that does not produce distractions or emphasize the configurations of the body.

1.5 In a mood of utmost seriousness and intensity, regulate the unlimited variables of bodily movement and posture through the authorized techniques of dancing, sitting, and moving the beads.

1.6 See to cleanliness, order, and symmetry of the external environment and physical body to foster a favorable mental environment for Sri Nama's appearance.

2.1 Offer obeisance to the spiritual master, the living example of pure hearing and chanting—the perfected mahamantra yogi.

2.2 Stabilize mental flux and turn consciousness inward by the brief exercise of establishing presence of self in the heart, regulating the breath, and focusing awareness on the inner field of vision.

2.3 Consider the gateways between the conscious self and the external world. These gateways are the five sensory systems.

2.4 Neglect the measuring and planning functions of the mind.

2.5 Residing in the organ of the heart as atomic sentience, lucidly visualize entrance into the four profound inner states described in the third verse of Sri Chaitanya Mahaprabhu's *Sri Sri Siksastaka*.

2.6 Complete the mental foundations for mahamantra yoga by firmly fixing the locus of awareness in the heart and meditating upon the Sri Panca-tattva mantra.

3.1 Produce the outward manifestation of Sri Nama Avatara by a vigorous coordinated effort of breath, vocal cords, jaw, tongue, and lips.

3.2 To sharpen enunciation of the mahamantra silently ask, "Who?"

3.3 While chanting and hearing the mahamantra, let breathing take care of itself.

3.4 While chanting and hearing the mahamantra, let speed be subservient to clear hearing.

3.5 While chanting and hearing the mahamantra let volume be subservient to clear hearing.

3.6 Let musical dimensions in mahamantra yoga play a minor, complementary, nondistracting role and nothing more.

4.1 Know Sri Nama Avatara to be the Supreme Person, the dynamic and vital Godhead, who directly acts within our life's course.

4.2 Know Sri Nama Avatara to be eternally spiritual—above material phenomena and distinct from all other sound vibrations.

4.3 Know Sri Nama Avatara as the primary reality in the superexcellent spiritual process for expansion of personal consciousness and realization of the ultimate truths of existence.

4.4 Know that the mahamantra is far more than His ephemeral shadow manifestation, which sincere neophyte practitioners usually experience. The real Sri Nama Avatara, the full manifestation of Godhead, is not invoked by a mere exercise of one's vocal mechanism. Rather, He descends through the agency of His pure devotees from the inconceivable plane of Goloka Vrindavana.

4.5 Know that Sri Nama Avatara is the gatekeeper—the resplendent regulator—of the expansion and contraction of one's personal consciousness.

4.6 Know that Sri Nama Avatara is the stupendously powerful agent who is ever eager to reveal, to those who love Him, limitless spiritual dimensions.

4.7 Know that the activity of hearing and chanting the mahamantra is our plea for engagement in spiritual service at the divine lotus feet of Sri Sri Radha Krishna, Who are the same as Sri Nama Avatara.

4.8 Know that by our hearing and chanting the mahamantra from the heart we invoke the presence of our supreme, intimate Friend—our Shelter, Benefactor, Director, Lord, and Purifier—Who appears before us as the incarnation of divine sound.

5.1 Now bring internal intensity to the foreground of consciousness.

5.2 Direct the mind's focus to the aural field.

5.3 Garland the mind with the third verse of Sri Chaitanya Mahaprabhu's *Sri Sri Siksastaka* and vividly feel the four states again and again.

5.4 As a baby cries for its mother, move consciousnesses to the heart and cry for the shelter of Sri Nama Avatara.

5.5 As one standing helplessly on death's threshold, continue to practice mahamantra yoga in a noncontrolling mood.

5.6 Feel strong love for Sri Nama Avatara—your savior.

5.7 Bathe your entire being in the purifying vibration of the mahamantra and directly perceive the resulting purification of your self.

5.8 Know that due to the powerful presence of Sri Nama Avatara you now mount the threshold of immense life-shattering and life-restructuring spiritual realizations.

5.9 Expel all traces of material egoism.

5.10 Expel all attitudes tending toward exploitation of Sri Nama Avatara such as desires for self-aggrandizement, sexual intercourse, and various other mundane pursuits.

5.11 Expel all thoughts of time, speed of recitation, numbers, and other calculative conceptions.

5.12 Expel all chanting methods that create distractions to mahamantra meditation.

5.13 Expel tendencies toward enjoyment of the new and wondrous inner domains of consciousness revealed by Sri Nama Avatara.

5.14 Expel all artificially forced mental approaches to Sri Nama Avatara: 1) By expressing deep faith in the mercy and potency of the mahamantra, and 2) By cultivating humility, devotion, service attitude, patience, reverence, and love.

6.1 That state of profound hearing and chanting of the mahamantra arises by the power and mercy of the mahamantra.

6.2 That state of profound hearing and chanting of the mahamantra is the dawning of the tireless stage of mahamantra meditation and practice.

6.3 That state of profound hearing and chanting of the mahamantra reveals all desires for self-aggrandizement and conquest of the world as utterly foolish and vain.

6.4 That state of profound hearing and chanting of the mahamantra is relished by the chanter in the way cool, sweet water is relished by a half-dead victim of the desert.

6.5 That state of profound hearing and chanting of the mahamantra engulfs and finally drowns the chanter by a powerful surge of nectar.

6.6 That state of profound hearing and chanting of the mahamantra causes the chanter to feel the inadequacy of his one tongue and two ears.

6.7 That state of profound hearing and chanting of the mahamantra thoroughly astounds the chanter.

6.8 Then the power and mercy of Sri Nama Avatara is ushered into the chanter's experience by Sri Nama Avatara Himself.

6.9 Then perceptions of the initial category of transcendence (brahman) are easily revealed through that power and mercy.

6.10 Then one becomes whole by Sri Nama Avatara's influence and realizes the pure spiritual self as well as utter distinction from all categories of material phenomena.

6.11 Then any doubts about the supreme reality of Sri Nama Avatara are destroyed at their roots.

6.12 Then Sri Nama Avatara—the realized form of the mahamantra—becomes the living, acting, directing, Godhead within one's life, bringing life into life.

6.13 Upon entering the internal forest by the profound hearing and chanting of the mahamantra, one falls flat before Him, knowing that He, Sri Nama Avatara, is the great shelter of all living beings.

6.14 Thus one gains powerful convictions and bold determinations to give the living mahamantra to others, to free them of the woes of phenomenal existence within matter.

6.15 All problems are rendered insignificant upon entering into the profound hearing and chanting of the mahamantra.

6.16 The mercy and ecstatic revelation of Sri Nama Avatara may be known sometimes even to neophyte chanters.

6.17 Upon reaching the internal forest by the path of profound hearing and chanting of the mahamantra, ecstatic transformations of the physical body occur spontaneously.

6.18 Upon reaching the internal forest by the path of profound hearing and chanting of the mahamantra one is unable to return to his birthplace, home, family, or society.

6.19 Upon reaching the internal forest by the profound hearing and chanting of the mahamantra all one's relative world conceptions meet with utter destruction.

6.20 The brilliant effulgence of Sri Nama Avatara is bursting through my small window! What is a window of light in comparison to the sun?

6.21 Oh fortunate living beings, hearers of the eternal glories of Sri Nama Avatara, know for certain that those glories are limitless! Indeed how much can atomic sentience say about Him? Here this tiny soul Sridhara dasa has minutely reflected the vast, illuminating, and extremely beautiful radiance of Sri Nama Avatara.

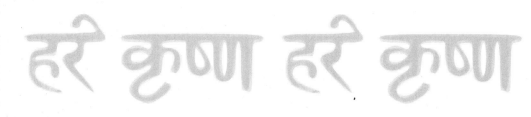

APPENDIX 3

*E*lucidations

Beacons of ascent to life's prime objective—perfection in mahamantra yoga.

Point 1. Follow in the footsteps of the previous mahamantra yogis—the perfected practitioners or acaryas.

Point 2. Become the menial servant of a genuine acarya of mahamantra yoga, receive the mahamantra from such a soul, and practically assist that great soul in the fulfillment of his or her vision.

Point 3. Become a knower of the sastras and a regular associate of sadhus, understanding both to be direct agents and expansions of Sri Nama Avatara.

Point 4. Follow the regulative principles of bhakti-yoga and know that Sri Nama Avatara realization is definitely accessible to that person who follows the authorized path.

Point 5. Communicate to interested persons the practice and glories of Sri Nama Avatara; you will thus develop and fix major thought programs for progressive mahamantra yoga within your mind as well as within the minds of others.

Point 6. Analyze and carefully control thought processes at all times.

Point 7. Know that thought control must ultimately be directed toward achieving the platform of unceasing, intensified focus of the mind upon the Supreme Absolute Person, Sri Sri Radha Krishna.

Point 8. Know that Krishna thought arouses spiritual taste, *bhakti-rasa.*

Point 9. Know that the initial stages of positive taste (*ruci*) experienced through some action is an essential element in creating further pursuance of that action.

Point 10. Know that the continual drive for taste, *rasa,* combined with a sincere spirit of philosophical inquiry, under the guidance of a pure devotee of Sri Sri Radha Krishna, delivers one to the plane of ceaseless chanting of the mahamantra.

Point 11. With care, regularly improve and purify the mental approach to ceaseless chanting of the mahamantra, and remember that ceaseless chanting is achieved by nurturing internal attitudes of service and humility.

Point 12. Develop the understanding that the Supreme Lord resides as the *Paramatma* (Supersoul) within the heart of every living being. Never consciously harm any living being and always live from the heart.

Point 13. Carefully control the urge to speak.

Point 14. Carefully avoid desires for material acquisition beyond what is needed.

Point 15. On the path of mahamantra yoga avoid unnecessary physical and mental distractions by:

> Eating only pure vegetarian *sattvic* foods that have been offered to the Supreme Lord
>
> Gradually reducing eating
>
> Resting sufficiently
>
> Carefully maintaining health

Point 16. Vanquish all taints of the ten offenses to Sri Nama Avatara.

Point 17. Make perfection of mahamantra yoga life's prime objective.

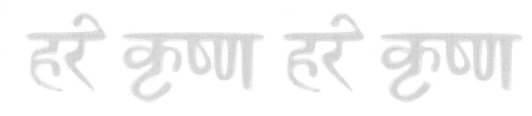

APPENDIX 4

*T*he Ten Offenses to the Holy Names

(From the *Padma Purana*)

1. *sadhu ninda:* criticism or harmful intent to a person qualified as *sadhu* or *Vaisnava.*
2. *sivasya sri-visnor ya iha guna-namadi-sakala dhiya bhinnam pasyet sa khalu hari-namahita-karah:* considering the names of demigods (such as Siva or Brahma or Kali) to be equal to or independent of the names of the *Visnu-tattva.*
3. *guru avajna:* disrespecting the guru and disobeying his orders.
4. *sruti-sastra-nindanam:* disrespecting the scriptural authority or blaspheming the Vedic literature (or literature in pursuance of the Vedic version).
5. *tatharthavado hari namni kalpanam:* thinking the glories of the mahamantra to be imaginary; giving some relative interpretation on the mahamantra.
6. *namno balad yasyahi papa buddhir:* committing sin on the strength of chanting the mahamantra.

7. *asraddadhane vimukhe'py asrnvati yas copadesah siva namaparadhah:* giving the instructions of mahamantra yoga to those who possess no faith or interest in the Lord or His transcendental name.

8. *dharma vrata tyaga hutadi sarve subha kriya samanyam ape pramadah:* considering the culture of mahamantra yoga to be on the same level as material pious activities.

9. *pramadah:* inattention or negligence while chanting the mahamantra.

10. *srute'pi nama mahatmye yah priti rahito' dhamah / aham mamadi paramonamni so'py aparadha krt:* not having complete faith in the mahamantra even after hearing from authorities about the greatness of the Name and maintaining material attachments by remaining obsessed with the conception of self and ownership—"It is I" and "It is mine."

हरे कृष्ण हरे कृष्ण

Bibliography

Titles marked with an asterisk (*) are books dealing with the science of bhakti-yoga to which the practice of mahamantra yoga belongs.

Aczel, Amir D. *The Mystery of the Aleph: Mathematics, the Kabbalah, and the Search for Infinity.* New York: Four Walls Eight Windows, 2000.

Andreas, Connirae. *Core Transformation.* Moab, Utah: Real People Press, 1994.

*Bhaktisiddhanta Saraswati Thakura. *Sri Brahma-Samhita.* Los Angeles, Calif.: Bhaktivedanta Book Trust International, 1985–2003.

———. *Sri Caitanya's Teachings.* Madras, India: Sri Gaudiya Math, 1973.

*Bhaktivedanta, A. C. (Swami Prabhupada). *Bhagavad-gita As It Is.* Los Angeles, Calif.: Bhaktivedanta Book Trust International, 1972–2004.

———. *Caitanya-caritamrta.* Los Angeles, Calif.: Bhaktivedanta Book Trust International, 1972–2003.

———. *The Nectar of Devotion.* Los Angeles, Calif.: Bhaktivedanta Book Trust International, 1969–2003.

———. *The Nectar of Instruction.* Los Angeles, Calif.: Bhaktivedanta Book Trust International, 1971–2003.

———. *Srimad-Bhagavatam.* Los Angeles, Calif.: Bhaktivedanta Book Trust International, 1972–2003.

———. *Teachings of Lord Kapila.* Los Angeles, Calif.: Bhaktivedanta Book Trust International, 1972–2003.

*Bhaktivinoda Thakura. *Jaiva Dharma.* Madras, India: Sri Gaudiya Math, 1975.

———. *Sri Chaitanya Mahaprabhu: His Life and Precepts.* Hooghly, West Bengal, India: Sri Gaudiya Vedanta Society, 1950.

———. *Sri Harinama-cintamani.* www.bvml.org/SBTP/hc.htm (2009).

———. *The Bhagavata: Its Philosophy, Its Ethics, and Its Theology.* www.bvml.org/SBTP/hc.htm (2009).

———. *Nama Bhajan.* www.bvml.org/SBTP/hc.htm. (2009).

*Bryant, Edwin F. *Krishna: The Beautiful Legend of God; Śrimad Bhāgavata Purāṇa, Book X.* London: Penguin Books, 2003.

———. *The Yoga Sūtras of Patañjali: A New Edition, Translation, and Commentary with Insights from the Traditional Commentators.* New York: North Point Press, 2009.

Buhner, Stephen Harrod. *The Secret Teachings of Plants.* Rochester, Vt.: Bear & Company, 2004.

Buxton, Simon. *The Shamanic Way of the Bee.* Rochester, Vt.: Destiny Books, 2004.

Castaneda, Carlos. *Journey to Ixtlan.* New York: Simon and Schuster, 1972.

Cohen, Michael J. *Reconnecting with Nature.* Corvallis, Ore.: Ecopress, 1997.

Conrad, Joseph. *Heart of Darkness and Other Stories.* London: CRW Publishing Ltd., 2006.

Croswell, Ken. *Magnificent Universe.* New York: Simon and Schuster, 1999.

Deikman, Arthur J. *The Observing Self: Mysticism and Psychotherapy.* Boston: Beacon Press, 1982.

Dilts, Robert, Tim Hallbom, and Suzi Smith. *Beliefs: Pathways to Health and Well-being.* Portland, Ore.: Metamorphous Press, 1990.

Gelberg, Steven J. *Hare Krishna, Hare Krishna: Five Distinguished Scholars on the Krishna Movement in the West.* New York: Grove Press, 1983.

Gillette, Douglas. *The Shaman's Secret: The Lost Resurrection Teachings of the Ancient Maya.* New York: Bantam Books, 1997.

Giono, Jean. *The Man Who Planted Trees.* London: Harvill Press, 1995.

Jaynes, Julian. *The Origin of Consciousness in the Breakdown of the Bicameral Mind.* Boston: Houghton Mifflin Company, 1990.

Johnson, Robert A. *Transformation: Understanding the Three Levels of Masculine Consciousness.* New York: HarperCollins Publishers, 1991.

Jung, C. G. Edited by Meredith Sabini. *The Earth Has a Soul: The Nature Writings of C. G. Jung.* Berkeley, Calif.: North Atlantic Books, 2002.

Kelley, Kevin W. *The Home Planet*. New York: Addison-Wesley Publishing Company, 1988.

Kingsley, Peter. *Reality*. Inverness, Calif.: The Golden Sufi Center, 2003.

Lauck, Joanne Elizabeth. *The Voice of the Infinite in the Small*. Boston: Shambhala Publications, Inc., 2002.

Lawlor, Robert. *Voices of the First Day: Awakening in the Aboriginal Dreamtime*. Rochester, Vt.: Inner Traditions International, 1991.

Lazaris. *The Sacred Journey: You and Your Higher Self*. Beverly Hills, Calif.: Concept: Synergy Publishing, 1987.

McKenna, Terence. *The Archaic Revival*. New York: HarperCollins Publishers, 1991.

Merton, Thomas. *Contemplative Prayer*. Garden City, N.Y.: Image Books, 1971.

Murchie, Guy. *The Seven Mysteries of Life*. London: Rider & Company, 1979.

Norris, Gunilla. *Inviting Silence*. London: Random House, 2005.

O'Donohue, John. *Divine Beauty: The Invisible Embrace*. London: Transworld/ Bantam Publishers, 2003.

Pearce, Joseph Chilton. *The Biology of Transcendence*. Rochester, Vt.: Park Street Press, 2002.

Rilke, Rainer Maria. *The Selected Poetry of Rainer Maria Rilke*. London: Pan Books Ltd., 1987.

Rossi, Ernest Lawrence. *The Psychobiology of Mind-Body Healing: New Concepts in Therapeutic Hypnosis*. New York: W. W. Norton & Co., 1993.

Sardello, Robert. *Facing the World with Soul*. Great Barrington, Mass.: Lindisfarne Press, 2004.

*Sridhara Deva Goswami (Srila Bhakti Raksaka). *Inner Fulfillment*. Nabadwip, India: Sri Caitanya Saraswat Math, 1995.

———. *Sri Guru and His Grace*. San Jose, Calif.: Guardian of Devotion Press, 1983.

———. *Subjective Evolution of Consciousness: The Play of the Sweet Absolute*. San Jose, Calif.: Guardian of Devotion Press, 1985.

———. *The Golden Volcano of Divine Love*. San Jose, Calif.: Guardian of Devotion Press, 1984.

———. *The Loving Search of the Lost Servant*. San Jose, Calif.: Guardian of Devotion Press, 1986.

————. *The Search for Sri Krishna: Reality the Beautiful*. San Jose, Calif.: Guardian of Devotion Press, 1983.

Stapledon, Olaf. *Star Maker*. London: Orion Publishing Group, 2003.

St. John of the Cross. *Dark Night of the Soul*. New York: Image Books, 1959.

Talbot, Michael. *The Holographic Universe*. London: HarperCollins Publishers, 1991.

Tarnas, Richard. *Cosmos and Psyche*. New York: Penguin Group, 2007.

Teilhard de Chardin, Pierre. *The Phenomena of Man*. London: William Collins Sons & Co., 1959.

Thoreau, Henry David. *Walden*. London: CRW Publishing Ltd., 2004.

Tolle, Eckhart. *A New Earth*. New York: Penguin Group Inc., 2005.

von Franz, Marie-Louise. *Alchemical Active Imagination*. Boston: Shambhala Publications, Inc., 1997.

Whitman, Walt. *Leaves of Grass*. New York: Penguin Books, 2005.

Wilber, Ken. *Sex, Ecology, Spirituality*. Boston: Shambhala Publications, Inc., 2000.

————. *The Spectrum of Consciousness*. Wheaton, Ill.: Theosophical Publishing House, 1993.

Wilson, Edward O. *The Diversity of Life*. Cambridge, Mass.: Belknap Press of Harvard University Press, 1992.

*I*ndex

How to Use This CD

This CD consists of three kirtans that were recorded live in Vrindaban, India. They are led by my dear godbrother His Grace Aindra Prabhu and are part of the twenty-four-hour kirtan program that has been going on at the Krishna-Balaram Mandir for more than twenty-five years. Here you will encounter an entire spectrum of the moods and the characteristics of authentic mahamantra yoga kirtan meditation.

The call-response style of these three kirtans is the group method taught by the realized mahamantra yogis, and it enables the participants to both hear and chant, thus focusing the mind between these two sensory arenas—the ears and the tongue. For the serious practitioner I suggest that you listen with either open-ear headphones or through conventional speakers. First hear Aindra leading the chant and then chant along with the group as it responds.

The various chapters of this book present the more detailed instruction for approaching your direct involvement in the mahamantra process. However, to briefly recap:

» Dis-identify from the physical body and the thinking mind.
» Assume the size of an atomic particle of pure consciousness situated within the heart.
» With eyes closed adopt an attitude of service and surrender to the most sublime aspects of the infinite personality of Godhead, Sri Sri Radha Krishna.
» In the mood of a baby crying out for its mother, cry out to mother Hara (Hare in the vocative), who is none other than Srimati Radharani.
» Ask for help from the perfected mahamantra yogis who have for hundreds of years worked tirelessly to deliver this process to humanity.

Readers may find out more about this twenty-four-hour non-stop program by visiting the website www.24hourkirtan.com. If you are contemplating a trip to India or live in India, you may participate in mahamantra yoga at the beautiful international-standards complex of the Krishna-Balaram Mandir founded in 1975 by His Divine Grace A. C. Bhaktivedanta Swami Prabhupada.